Gastrointestinal Motility

TO RUTH, JOE AND RICHARD

Gastrointestinal Motility
The Integration of Physiological Mechanisms

By David Grundy

Lecturer in Physiology, University of Sheffield

MTP PRESS LIMITED
a member of the KLUWER ACADEMIC PUBLISHERS GROUP
LANCASTER / BOSTON / THE HAGUE / DORDRECHT

Published in the UK by
MTP Press Limited
Falcon House
Lancaster, England

British Library Cataloguing in Publication Data
Grundy, David
  Gastrointestinal motility: the integration of physiological mechanisms.
  1. Gastrointestinal system—Motility
  I. Title
612′.32   QP180

ISBN-13: 978-94-010-9357-6   e-ISBN-13: 978-94-010-9355-2
DOI: 10.1007/978-94-010-9355-2

Published in the USA by
MTP Press
A division of Kluwer Boston Inc
190 Old Derby Street
Hingham, MA 02043, USA

Library of Congress Cataloging in Publication Data
Grundy, David.
  Gastrointestinal motility.

  Bibliography: p.
  Includes index.
  1. Gastrointestinal system—Motility.   2. Peristalsis.
  I. Title. [DNLM: 1. Gastrointestinal Motility.
  WI 102 G889g]
  QP180.G78 1985   599′.0132   85–7189

  ISBN-13: 978-94-010-9357-6

Phototypesetting by Titus Wilson, Kendal, Cumbria, England

Tiptree, Essex

Contents

Contents

Preface

The basis of this book is a ten-lecture course on the control of gastrointestinal motility given each year to the final year undergraduate students in Physiology at Sheffield University. A naive thought led me to believe that the conversion of my lecture notes into the present book would be a relatively easy task. I now know differently.

As there is no equivalent undergraduate course elsewhere that I know of, it would be dishonest of me to claim this book to be an undergraduate text. The comprehensive way in which I have dealt with the subject, together with the inclusion of the most up-to-date material, make the book more relevant to postgraduate students of physiology, medicine and related sciences who require an introduction to the field of gastrointestinal motility and its control. I have, however, attempted to present the current concepts on the physiological mechanisms regulating motility in a way which undergraduates, as well as postgraduates, will find readable, informative and, hopefully, enjoyable.

I have concentrated on the control of normal motor function and commented on malfunction only when it gives insight into the underlying physiological mechanisms. However, it should be apparent to all that a sound understanding of physiology is a prerequisite for the interpretation of the diseased state. The emphasis is on human gastrointestinal motility but the need for suitable animal models in order to elucidate the control mechanisms means that much of the experimental evidence described in this book relates to species other than man. There is a little comparative physiology but, unless otherwise stated, the concepts for control developed in other animals are probably also applicable to man.

As readability was high on my list of priorities I have avoided making the text an exhaustive list of references. Where possible, review articles are quoted that will provide the reader with a reference source from which to assess the literature. To complement this approach a two-tier bibliography is provided. A book list provides a guide to further reading, while in addition there is a complete list of all references either quoted in the text or used as a source of illustrations. Many of these are recent papers that have not yet found their way into reviews. I am grateful to all those who have allowed me to use their illustrations and especially so to those who have provided copies of original photographs.

I have taken as my definition of the gastrointestinal tract the straight-line approach and considered only the viscera connecting the pharynx and anus. The content of the book builds from properties of smooth muscle cells and their regulation by intrinsic and extrinsic influences, through the control of individual regions and finally considers the system as a whole. The book concentrates on control processes and I make no apology for the emphasis on neural rather than hormonal mechanisms – this is not to say that hormones are less important in the regulatory processes but this merely reflects my own interest in the autonomic nervous system.

David Grundy

1
Gastrointestinal smooth muscle

INTRODUCTION

The contractions and relaxations of gastrointestinal smooth muscle are essential for maintaining the orderly process of digestion. The progress of gastrointestinal contents along the gut is matched to the volume and composition of food ingested and the rate of its subsequent modification by digestion and absorption. Inhibition of spontaneous tone allows smooth muscle cells to relax thereby enabling sphincters to open or digesta to be accommodated in regions like the stomach. Contractions, on the other hand, provide the propulsive force which moves digesta along the gastrointestinal tract, and additionally ensures adequate mixing of ingested material with digestive enzymes, and continuously brings nutrients into contact with the absorptive mucosal surface.

The energy for contraction is, like that in skeletal and cardiac muscle, derived from the hydrolysis of adenosine triphosphate (ATP). In this way chemical energy is converted to mechanical energy causing the muscle cells to either shorten or develop tension. This cellular event is the endpoint of a complex chain of events whereby the behaviour of the muscle is subjected to a hierarchical arrangement of controls from external nervous and hormonal influences. However, the basis for all gastrointestinal motility is the muscle's own ability to generate cyclical changes in its resting membrane potential which, if conditions are right, give rise to spontaneous, rhythmical contractions. Thus, a feature of visceral smooth muscle that has fascinated scientists for centuries is the rhythmic motility seen in segments of the gastrointestinal tract totally removed from the body. In this chapter the organization and properties of smooth muscle that provide the basis for myogenic contractions are described.

SMOOTH MUSCLE CELLS

Smooth muscle cells are small mononucleate cells. They are often considered to be spindle-shaped but in reality vary considerably and are much more irregularly shaped. At rest the muscle cells are between 500 and 700 μm in length and approximately 5 μm in diameter and are orientated so that their long axes run in one direction. In most regions of the gastrointestinal tract two layers of smooth muscle can be distinguished

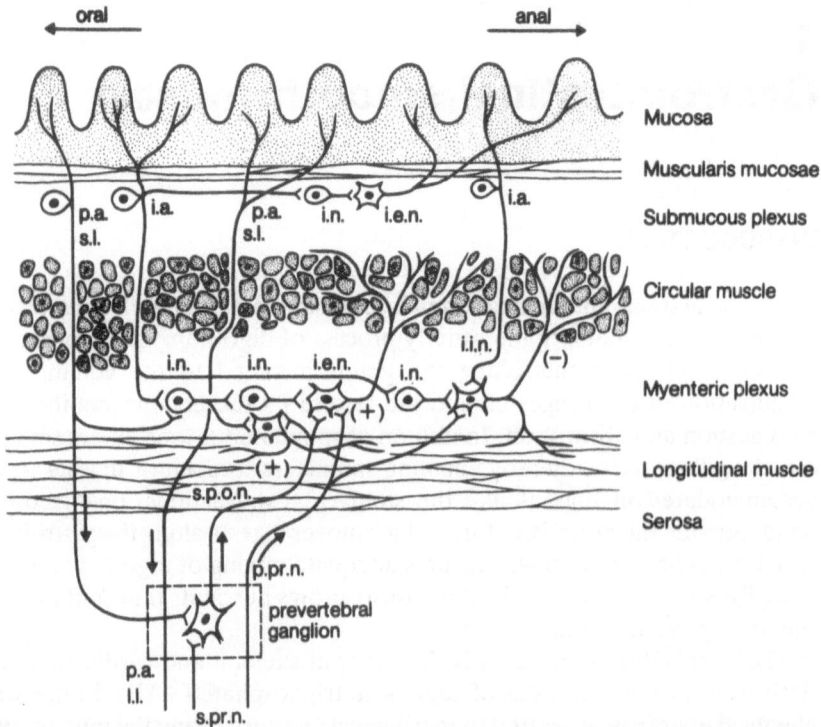

Figure 1.1 Schematic portrayal of the bowel wall and its extrinsic innervation. The longitudinal and circular muscle layers are evident as are the two nerve plexuses which innervate them. Symbols: + = excitatory; — = inhibitory; i.a. = intrinsic afferent; p.a.s.l. = primary afferent short loop; p.a.l.l. = promary afferent long loop; i.n. = interneurone; i.e.n. = intrinsic excitatory neurone; i.i.n = intrinsic inhibitory neurone; s.pr.n. = sympathetic preganglionic nerve; p.pr.n. = parasympathetic preganglionic nerve (From Baumgarten, 1982, with kind permission of the author and publisher, Springer–Verlag)

from the adjacent nerve plexuses and mucosal tissue (Figure 1.1). Cells in the outer coat of smooth muscle are orientated to run longitudinally, while muscle cells in the inner layer run circumferentially. Only in the stomach is there a third, oblique, layer of muscle but this is incomplete and consists merely of two bands of muscle running along the anterior and posterior surfaces of the stomach. A thin layer of muscle in the submucosae regulates the movements of the mucosa during digestion, but has no effect on the bulk movement of luminal contents and will not be discussed further.

Skeletal muscle cells are many times the size of smooth muscle cells

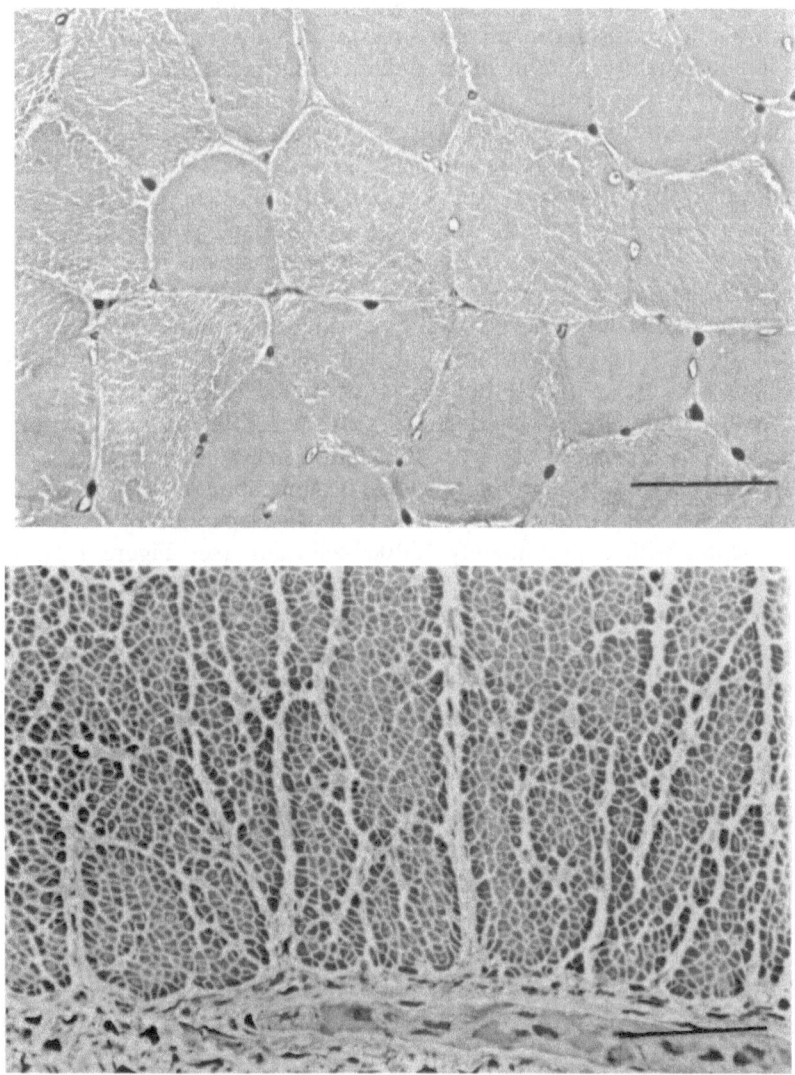

Figure 1.2 Transverse section through guinea-pig satorius muscle (upper) and taenia coli (lower) examined unstained in phase-contrast microscopy. Bar: $50\,\mu$m (From Gabella, 1979a, with kind permission of the author and editor of Br. Med. Bull.)

(Figure 1.2). Consequently, the latter have a very large surface area-to-volume ratio. This causes problems in maintaining intracellular ionic content since the sarcoplasm is always in close proximity to the cell membrane where the potential for ionic exchange exists, and there is no large bulk of sarcoplasm within which small changes in ionic composition can be buffered. To counteract this, the membrane resistance per unit area is approximately five times higher in smooth compared to skeletal muscle cells. This high resistance is due to a reduced passive permeability to ions which reduces fluctuations in intracellular ions and allows ionic composition to be maintained without expending an excessive amount of energy in the expulsion of unwanted ions. However, because smooth muscle cells are seldom totally at rest due to their intrinsic rhythmicity and continuous bombardment with neurotransmitters and hormones, none of the major ions are in equilibrium with the resting membrane potential. Smooth muscle cells, therefore, have well-developed mechanisms for transporting ions and for maintaining a constant intracellular environment. Of particular importance is the machinery which limits the intracellular concentration of calcium ions since, as with all other muscles, Ca^{2+} ions provide the mechanism whereby muscle tension is controlled. Therefore, there is a membrane bound Na–Ca exchange pump and an ATP-dependent Ca pump which actively extrudes Ca^{2+} from the resting smooth muscle cells.

Another feature of smooth muscle cells brought about by their small size is their organization into densely packed bundles, separated by connective tissue septa, with approximately 180 000 cells/mm³ (see Figure 1.2). Of paramount importance for this arrangement is the structure of surface junctions between adjacent cells which allow individual cells to cooperate both electrically and mechanically. It is because of this coupling between adjacent cells that the functional unit for gastrointestinal contractions is considered to be a bundle of smooth muscle cells with individual cells forming part of a three-dimensional syncytium. Each cell is separated from its neighbour by a gap of about 60 nm filled with basement membrane material. However, there are specialized regions of cell membrane where the gap is much less and where intimate contact between adjacent cells is made. These provide the basis for mechanical and electrical coupling.

Dense bands

Viewed under an electron microscope, 50% of the membrane of smooth muscle cells appears to be covered with regions where electron-dense material is firmly encrusted on the inner membrane surface (Figure 1.3). Actin filaments, one of the basic contractile proteins, penetrate the dense bands and are firmly anchored there. These dense bands are therefore the equivalent of the Z-bands of striated muscle (readers who are unfamiliar with the structure of striated muscle and the sliding filament theory of contraction should see Wilkie, 1976). Since dense bands occur periodically over the entire cell membrane and are not rigidly ordered as in striated muscle, smooth muscle cells appear smooth when viewed through the light microscope as compared with the striated skeletal muscle. Dense bands can also occur more deeply in the sarcoplasm.

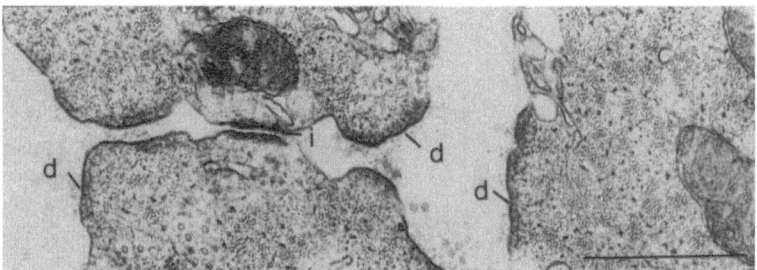

Figure 1.3 Transverse section of guinea-pig taenia coli. Bar; 1 μm. Symbols: d = dense bands; i = intermediate junction (From Gabella, 1979a, with kind permission of the author and editor of Br. Med. Bull.)

Intermediate junctions

Dense bands on adjacent cells are often matched in structure and size. Where these occur they form a symmetrical junction, 1–2 μm in length, known as an intermediate junction. The cleft between the adjacent cells is 30–40nm and while there is no cytoplasmic continuity the region is held together by an electron-dense intercellular cement (see Figure 1.3). These intermediate junctions are the site of mechanical coupling between smooth muscle cells and they provide a direct link between the contractile unit of one cell and its neighbour. Where dense bands occur outside intermediate junctions they are seen to be anchored to collagen fibrils which are abundant in the intracellular space. These anchorage points are necessary for movement of the cell as a whole and not just within the cytoplasm. The collagen can therefore be considered as intramuscular tendons.

Gap junctions

A second type of junction associated with some types of smooth muscle is the nexus or gap junction. At these junctions adjacent cells come into very close proximity with only a 2–3 nm gap between them (Figure 1.4). Studies using intracellular dyes show that this gap is bridged by channels that allow ions and small molecules to pass from one cell to the next. Gap junctions are therefore considered to be the sites for electrical coupling between cells. A measure of the degree of this coupling can be obtained by measuring the spread of current through the smooth muscle mass (Albe and Tomita, 1968). Strips of smooth muscle are passed through polarizing plates. An intracellular microelectrode is then used to measure the potential changes in cells at a distance from the plates. The electrotonic potential is found to decay exponentially with distance and is characterized in different tissues by the 'space constant'. This is defined as the distance over which the potential falls to 1/e of its original value and increases as the resistance between cells decreases. Values for the space constant are greatest in the direction of the long axes of the cells and typical values vary between 1

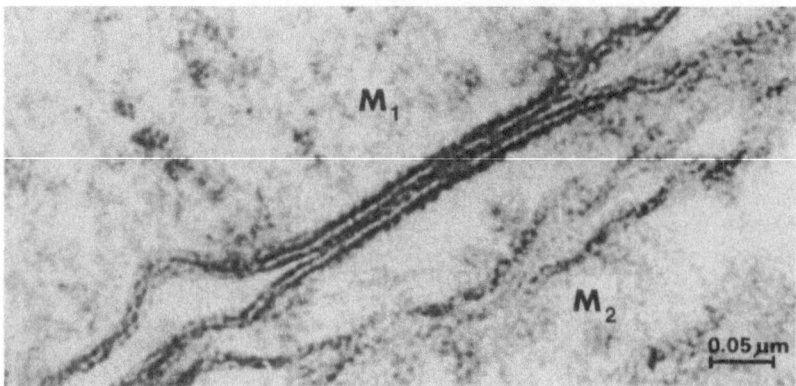

Figure 1.4 Gap junction between two smooth muscle cells grown in tissue culture. Magnification 196 000×. Reproduced with kind permission of the authors and *The Journal of Cell Biology* (1971), **49**, pp. 21-34 by copyright permission of The Rockefeller University Press

and 3 mm which is considerably longer than the length of individual cells. Electrical activity, therefore, spreads from one cell to the next through low resistant pathways. However, although gap junctions are abundant in the circular muscle layer they are absent in the longitudinal muscle layer. While this supports the observation that there is less electrical interaction between longitudinal muscle cells, longitudinal muscle nevertheless shows good electrical coupling. There must, therefore, be other structures that electrically couple longitudinal muscle cells which have yet to be characterized.

CONTRACTILE SYSTEM

The contractile system is basically the same in smooth muscle as that studied in more detail in skeletal muscle. The contractile proteins actin and myosin are both present in smooth muscle and the sliding filament theory for muscle contraction whereby active shortening is caused by the movement of cross-bridges formed between the actin and myosin filaments still holds. There are, however, several differences between skeletal and smooth muscle with regard to the way interactions between actin and myosin are regulated. When pure actin and myosin, extracted from skeletal muscle, are mixed in a test tube they form a complex called actomyosin. In normal resting muscle this active state is inhibited due to the presence of the regulatory protein complex, troponin–tropomyosin, on the actin filament. The trigger for contraction is an elevation of intracellular calcium brought about by depolarization of the muscle cell. The Ca^{2+} binds to troponin and brings about a conformational change allowing actin and myosin to form cross-bridges which repeatedly pivot with hydrolysis of ATP causing the actin and myosin to slide over each other.

Actin and myosin extracted from smooth muscle will not react when mixed together (Hartshorne, 1981). Unlike the case in skeletal muscle, actin and myosin from smooth muscle exists in a dormant state which only becomes active when there is a rise in intracellular Ca^{2+} ion concentration. Regulation of the active state in smooth muscle is brought about by an enzyme which phosphorylates part of the myosin cross-bridge. The enzyme, myosin light-chain kinase, has two subunits –one being the enzyme proper and the other a calcium-binding protein, calmodulin. Thus calcium binds to calmodulin which activates the enzyme to phosphorylate the myosin cross-bridges. Only when phosphorylated will actin and myosin interact, repeated cycles of actin-mediated ATP hydrolysis–cross-bridge formation then continue and the muscle shortens or develops tension. The sequence is terminated when the sarcoplasmic calcium ion concentration is returned to below 10^{-7} mol/l and the kinase deactivated. A second enzyme, myosin light chain phosphatase, removes the phosphate from the myosin cross-bridge which returns the myosin to its inactive state and relaxation follows. In both skeletal and smooth muscle, therefore, an increase in sarcoplasmic calcium ion concentration is a prerequisite for contraction but the mechanism by which calcium brings about this contraction is quite different (Table 1.1).

Table 1.1 Summary of the contractile process in skeletal and smooth muscle

	Striated muscle	Smooth muscle
Contractile proteins	Acton and myosin held in restraint by tropinin/tropomyosin (TT) complex	Dormant actin and myosin
Trigger	Calcium ions	Calcium ions
Target protein	Troponin	Calmodulin
Effect	Conformational change in TT complex	Phosphorylation of myosin cross-bridge
Result	Cross-bridges formed	Cross-bridges formed
Terminated by	Removal of calcium	Removal of calcium
Effect	TT complex again inhibits actomyosin formation	Myosin dephosphorylated; returns to dormant state

Another difference between skeletal and smooth muscle is the source of Ca^{2+} for triggering contraction. In both tissues a rise in sarcoplasmic Ca^{2+} from resting levels of about 10^{-7} mol/l up to between 1 and 10 μmol/l is the trigger for contraction. The source of this Ca^{2+}, however, is different. In skeletal muscle there is an extensive sarcoplasmic reticulum constituting 20% of the dry weight of the cells. Ca^{2+} is stored in the terminal cisternae of this sarcoplasmic reticulum and is released when an action potential propagates through the muscle. In smooth muscle, only 1–2% of the dry weight of the cells is sarcoplasmic reticulum. Other sources of calcium may reside in the mitochondria and it is calculated that there is sufficient Ca^{2+} in intracellular stores to provide the coupling between the cell action potential and the muscle contraction. However, contractions of smooth muscle are rapidly lost when extracellular Ca^{2+} is removed. This suggests that extracellular Ca^{2+} is important for either filling the intracellular stores, causing their release, or, as we shall see below, directly activating the contractile apparatus.

Smooth muscle can shorten to a greater extent than skeletal muscle. Maximally contracted smooth muscle cells can be less than one-quarter of their original resting length. Smooth muscle cells can also contract when stretched to a greater extent than skeletal muscle, a property that is important for organs like the stomach. This may be as a consequence of the less rigid arrangement of contractile filaments (Figure 1.5).

(A)   (B)

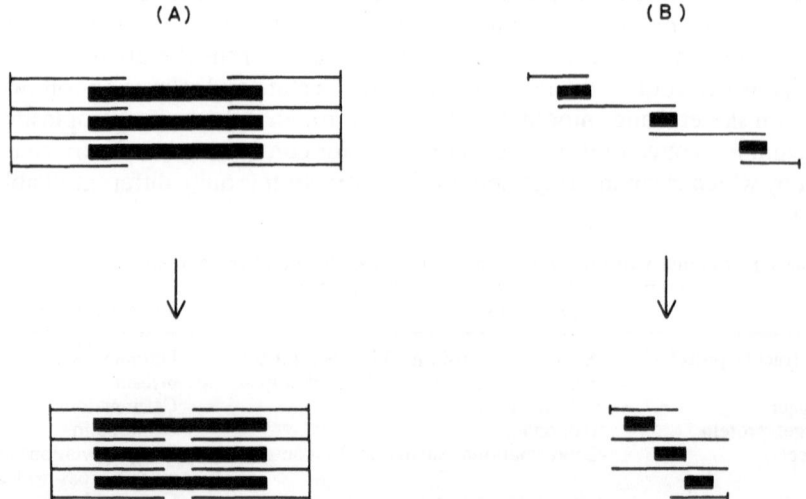

Figure 1.5 Arrangement of myosin (thick filaments) and actin (thin filaments) in skeletal (A) and smooth (B) muscle during shortening (Adapted from Aidley, 1978, and Small and Squire, 1972)

Aiding these considerable changes in cell shape are caveolae on the cell membrane. These are flask-shaped invaginations of the cell membrane measuring about 70 nm in diameter (Figure 1.6). They occur in the region of membrane devoid of dense bands and are calculated to increase the surface area by approximately 70%. During shortening, the cell membrane undergoes remarkable changes. The region of membrane containing caveolae can fold giving the membrane a corrugated appearance. The folds from adjacent cells interdigitate allowing the cells to considerably shorten in length. In the opposite direction, stretching causes the cell membranes to become smooth. One suggestion for the ability of smooth muscle cells to

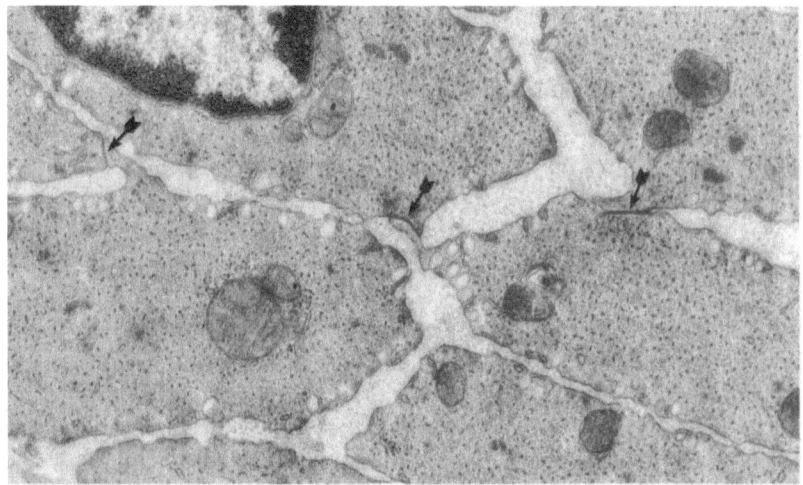

Figure 1.6 Circular muscle of rat ileum. Three gap junctions are marked by arrows. Note also caveolae in cell membrane. Magnification 15000× (From Gabella, 1981, with kind permission of the author and publisher, Raven Press)

be greatly stretched is that the caveolae open out. While this has been observed in some invertebrate smooth muscle, the number of caveolae and the diameter of their necks in visceral smooth muscle is unaffected by even severe stretching.

Another possible role for caveolae is as an extracellular store for calcium since they appear in close proximity to the sarcoplasmic reticulum.

ELECTRICAL PROPERTIES OF SMOOTH MUSCLE CELLS

Resting membrane potential

The low permeability of the smooth muscle cell membrane, mentioned briefly above, helps maintain a relatively constant internal ionic environment. However, from Table 1.2 one can see that there are considerable differences between the internal and external ionic concentrations of the major ions which carry current across the cell membrane. The values for the internal concentrations are calculated from the total ion content of smooth muscle tissue, corrected for the volume and composition of the extracellular fluid and intracellular compartments. There are considerable technical difficulties associated with the assessment of the extracellular volume because of the small smooth muscle cells being densely packed and therefore not readily accessible to extracellular markers such as inulin and sorbitol. The values in Table 1.2 are therefore approximations.

In the absence of an electrical potential across the membrane, these

Table 1.2 Internal and external concentration of the major current carrying ions in intestinal smooth muscle and their equilibrium potentials calculated from the Nernst equation (data from Bortoff, 1983)

	Internal concentration (mmol/l)	External concentration (mmol/l)	Equilibrium potential (mV)
K	164	5	−91
Na	13	140	62
Cl⁻	58	134	−22
Ca²	0.0001	1.8	>120

ions would move across the membrane at a rate proportional to the concentration gradient and the permeability of the membrane to each ion. Thus, potassium ions, being the most permeable, would diffuse out of the cell. However, the presence of a resting membrane potential, the inside of the cell being negative relative to the outside, would tend to attract positively charged potassium ions. This would reduce the loss of potassium from the cell or, if the potential difference is large enough, reverse the flow of potassium ions. The algebraic sum of these two forces is called the electrochemical potential gradient and determines the net flow of ions across the membrane. If the electrochemical gradient is zero, the chemical gradient is exactly matched by the opposite electrical gradient, there is no net movement of ions and eqilibrium conditions are achieved. The membrane potential at equilibrium for a particular ion can therefore be calculated by equating the electrical potential attracting ions in one direction and the opposing chemical gradient. Thus:

$$\text{electrical force} = ZFE$$

where
$$Z = \text{ion valency}$$
$$F = \text{the Faraday constant}$$
$$E = \text{potential difference}$$

and

$$\text{chemical force} = RT \ln \frac{[C] \text{ outside}}{[C] \text{ inside}}$$

where
$$R = \text{gas constant}$$
$$T = \text{absolute temperature}$$
$$\ln = \text{natural logarithm}$$
$$C = \text{ionic concentration}$$

At equilibrium these two forces are equal and opposite; equating the two and solving for E gives the Nernst equation:

$$E = \frac{RT}{ZF} \ln \frac{[C] \text{ outside}}{[C] \text{ inside}}$$

The equilibrium potentials for the major ions calculated from the Nernst equation is shown in Table 1.2.

The resting membrane potentials of smooth muscle cells from different regions of the gastrointestinal tract have been investigated using microelectrodes inserted directly into the cells, although this technique is difficult because of the small size of the cells. Nevertheless experimental values generally vary between -40 and $-75\,mV$. Comparing these recorded values with the calculated equilibrium potentials in Table 1.2 it can be seen that none of the major ions are in equilibrium with the membrane potential and therefore none are distributed entirely by passive forces. Under these circumstances the net movement of a particular ion is determined by the difference between the actual membrane potential and the ion's equilibrium potential. Thus at the resting membrane potential the cell would lose potassium ions and accumulate sodium ions. This is counteracted by a sodium–potassium exchange pump on the cell membrane. This pump accumulates potassium inside the cell and at the same time keeps the internal sodium concentration low. However, the number of sodium and potassium ions exchanged are not equal, three sodium ions being pumped out of the cell for every two potassium ions pumped in. A net positive charge is therefore carried from the inside of the cell, and thus hyperpolarizes the membrane making the inside more negative. The pump is called 'electrogenic' because it contributes directly to the negative intracellular potential. Active mechanisms must also be responsible for elevating the internal Cl^- ion concentration above the level that would be expected from its passive distribution. Cl^- ions become passively distributed when the sodium–potassium pump is blocked indicating a link between the transport of all these ions.

Resting membrane potentials calculated on the basis of all the contributing ions and their relative permeabilities generally give values less negative than the experimental data (Casteels, 1969). The difference between the two probably reflects the contribution from the electrogenic pump although the precise contribution from the latter is controversial and estimates vary between 4 and $20\,mV$.

Slow waves

Having established a basis for the resting membrane potential in gastrointestinal smooth muscle, one needs to modify this slightly to account for the inherent rhythmicity seen in some visceral smooth muscle cells. Smooth muscle from the longitudinal muscle layer of the small intestine or circular muscle layer of the stomach and colon generate rhythmic, spontaneous depolarization. These periodic fluctuations in the resting membrane potential are called slow waves because of the low frequency of the oscillations. The actual frequency of the slow wave varies between different regions of the gastrointestinal tract and shows species differences. In man they occur at approximately 3/min in the stomach and 12/min in the duodenum. Slow waves have also been termed: basic electrical rhythm (BER) because they are always present even when there is no contractile activity; pacemaker potentials because they determine the maximum frequency of muscle contractions; and electrical control activity (ECA) because of the way they control contractions. Individual cells exist in a syncytium and hence show synchronous slow wave activity with the highest slow wave frequency acting as a pacemaker. In this way the slow wave frequency at any one point is influenced by slow waves from adjacent regions so that the slow wave appears to propagate through the muscle mass at a velocity determined by the degree of electrical coupling (see p. 119).

The slow wave recorded with intracellular electrodes appears as a low amplitude, monophasic depolarization consisting of an initial rapid depolarization followed by a plateau with a slow repolarization (Figure

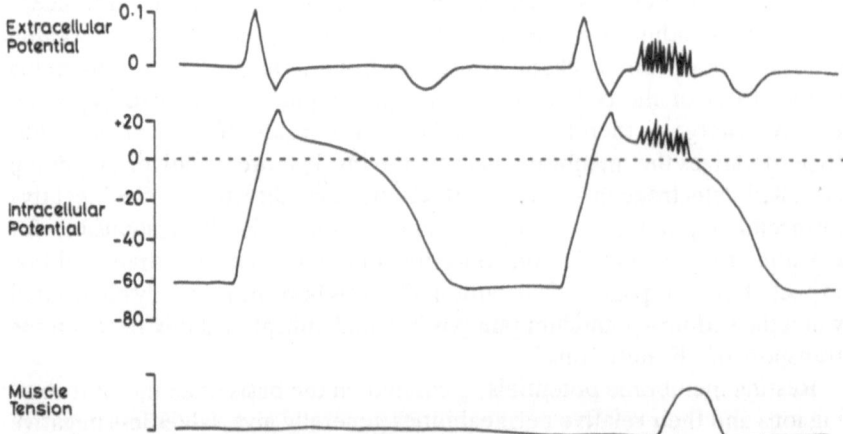

Figure 1.7 Schematic representation of the relationship between electrical potentials recorded with intracellular and extracellular electrodes. On the right action potentials occur during the plateau phase of the slow wave (shown without action potentials on the left) and result in contraction of the muscle (Adapted from Caprilli, Frieri and Vernia, 1982)

1.7). Two hypotheses have been put forward to explain the ionic basis of the slow wave. The first suggests that the slow wave is due to cyclical variations in the membrane permeability to sodium ions and as such requires a critical concentration of sodium ions in the extracellular medium. Reducing the sodium ion concentration below this reduces or abolishes the slow waves. Thus an increase in the sodium ion permeability would give rise to the depolarization phase of the slow wave. The second hypothesis proposes oscillatory activity of the electrogenic Na–K pump. Depolarization would occur if the activity of the pump was suppressed temporarily while switching the pump back on would hyperpolarize the membrane to its original level. Several pieces of evidence support this latter hypothesis:

(1) Activity of the pump requires potassium in the extracellular fluid. Removing this or treating the muscle with ouabain, a glycoside extracted from certain plants, inhibits the pump and also abolishes the slow wave.

(2) The efflux of a radioisotope of sodium (^{24}Na) from smooth muscle cells can be followed after previously loading the cells with this isotope. In these experiments the efflux peaks at the beginning of the repolarization phase suggesting that Na–K pump activity is maximal at this point in time.

(3) During the application of voltage clamp to strips of smooth muscle, a technique whereby the membrane potential is held constant at any particular level while current flow through the membrane is measured, there is a transient inward current at the same frequency as the slow wave.

(4) The activity of the pump requires energy derived from ATP. Metabolic inhibitors like 2,4-dinitrophenol or cyanide which remove the energy source also block the slow waves.

This evidence implies an important role for sodium extrusion by the electrogenic Na–K pump in the genesis of slow waves. However, the ionic mechanism may not necessarily be the same in all gastrointestinal smooth muscle.

Action potentials

The slow waves described above do not initiate contractions of the muscle but represent cyclical changes in smooth muscle excitability. They do, however, play an important part in determining when contractions can occur by bringing the resting membrane potential near to the threshold for the generation of action potentials. When the threshold is reached, voltage-dependent channels in the membrane are opened giving rise to the ionic movements responsible for the generation of action potentials. The amplitude of individual action potentials are not constant, as with the 'all or none' action potential in nerve and skeletal muscle, but have variable amplitudes (see Figure 1.7). The amplitude of the evoked contraction is determined by the number of action potentials superimposed on each slow wave.

The action potential in smooth muscle shows other differences from those described in nerve and skeletal muscle. Firstly, the spikes are much slower with a rise time of 5–20 V s^{-1} (compare 1000 V s^{-1} in skeletal muscle) and have a longer duration of 7–20 ms. Because of the relative slowness of these action potentials they are often referred to as spikes.

Unlike those in nerve and skeletal muscle, smooth muscle action potentials are resistant to treatment with tetrodotoxin (puffer fish venom) wich selectively blocks voltage-dependent sodium channels. The inward current

13

of the action potential is therefore not carried by sodium ions but is blocked by interference with the entry of calcium into the cell. Thus, replacing Ca^{2+} with Mg^{2+} in the extracellular fluid or treating with a calcium channel blocker (verapamil) blocks the action potentials. The action potential in smooth muscle therefore depends mainly if not exclusively on the inward movement of Ca^{2+} ions that are believed to be either bound to the extracellular membrane or stored within the caveolae, since the rundown of action potentials after the removal of all extracellular calcium ions takes several minutes.

Calcium therefore carries the inward current and provides a direct coupling of the contractile mechanism with electrical events. Calcium action potentials would be inappropriate in nerves where rapid transmission is essential, but in smooth muscle it is not disadvantageous to the slowly moving visceral organs. The calcium entry during the action potential is fast enough for smooth muscle contractions so that there is no need for the rapid release mechanism of the sarcoplasmic reticulum in skeletal muscle.

The repolarization phase of the smooth muscle action potentials depends on the opening of voltage dependent potassium channels in much the same way as in nerve and skeletal muscle. But unlike the situation in nerves, where sodium provides a fast inward current, the slow inward Ca^{2+} current and the outward K^+ current have similar time-courses. The increased potassium conductance, therefore, limits the peak potential of the spike and makes its amplitude more variable. Treating the membrane with a potassium channel blocker like tetraethylammonium converts the variable action potentials to a more regular 'all or none' spike.

The smooth muscle spike or action potential therefore depends upon a different ionic mechanism from that of nerves. This provides a means of selectively blocking nervous conduction using tetrodotoxin without affecting smooth muscle contractions, and provides a useful means of chemically denervating muscle (see p. 18).

In gastric smooth muscle, action potentials are not a prerequisite for contractions. Instead, the slow waves are followed by a plateau potential whose amplitude and duration determine the magnitude of the contractions (see Chapter 6).

Smooth muscle syncytium

Slow waves recorded from closely spaced electrodes appear to propagate from the region with the highest intrinsic frequency. The membrane currents associated with spike activity also pass outwards to other cells through low-resistant pathways. Since contractions develop when the slow wave reaches the threshold for action potential the direction and velocity at which the contraction propagate are both determined by the slow wave. The circular muscle is closely coupled ensuring that a ring of contraction develops almost simultaneously around the full circumference of the viscera. The longitudinal muscle is less well coupled. Here, action potentials propagate more slowly and provide the basis for peristalsis whereby a ring of circular muscle contraction propagates a short distance along the gastrointestinal tract. The bundle of smooth muscle is therefore the functional unit of gastrointestinal contractions. This point is emphasized in the way single smooth muscle cells respond to the injection of depolarizing currents through a microelectrode. The current rapidly dissipates as it flows outwards through the low-resistant pathways and thus the membrane potential seldom reaches threshold for spike generation (Holman and Neild, 1979). Only when many cells are synchronously activitated, for example by stimulation through plate electrodes or by the exogenous application of acetylcholine, does depolarization reach the threshold for spike activity and contractions follow.

Extracellular correlates of intracellular events

Since slow waves and spikes occur synchronously in many cells they can be detected on the serosal surface of the gut wall with large extracellular electrodes. Alvarez and Mahoney (1922) recorded continuous 'action currents' from the serosal surface irrespective of whether contractions were present or not. These are the extracellular correlates of slow wave activity. Contractions were later seen to be associated with more rapid changes in potential which were superimposed on the slow wave oscillations (Bozler, 1939). This relationship between spikes and contractions allows indirect recordings of contractile activity to be made from the serosal surface without interfering with the continuity of the gut wall (see Figure 1.7). The occurrence of spikes is taken to represent contractile activity while the number of spikes on each slow wave gives an indication of the force of contraction. This type of data is commonly quantified in either of two ways: as a percentage of slow waves that also carry spikes or as the total number of spikes per unit time. This electromyographic technique is one of the most important methods employed in the study of gastrointestinal motility today and has undoubtedly contributed greatly to our present knowledge of motor function.

EXTERNAL INFLUENCES ON SMOOTH MUSCLE

Chemical recognition sites on the smooth muscle cell membrane are the means by which the muscle's myogenic properties are regulated. Receptors to a variety of neurotransmitters and hormones mediate contraction and relaxation either by altering the various features of the membrane potential or by modifying enzyme systems involved in the contractile process. Excitation can be produced in several ways. Membrane depolarization resulting from a general increase in membrane permeability or the increase in permeability to specific ions will take the membrane potential nearer the threshold for spikes which may occur as the slow wave depolarizes the cell membrane further. This may initiate contractions if none are present or increase the amplitude of any existing contractions. Similar effects will result from an increase in the amplitude of the slow waves or a lowering of the threshold for spike generation. Contractions would also be achieved by the release of internal calcium stores or by increasing the activity of the phosphorylating enzymes regulating the interaction of actin and myosin. Inhibition could result from the opposite of any of the above.

This is not an exhaustive list and many endogenous substances such as acetylcholine and noradrenaline exert their effects through a combination of the above (see Daniel, 1982). However, the final outcome of any regulatory mechanism must always be the same – that is the modification of interactions between the contractile proteins.

2
Intramural ganglia and mechanism of peristalsis

INTRODUCTION

Whole segments of the gastrointestinal tract when removed from the body and maintained in physiological solutions can perform complex and coordinated contractile activity. The basis for this is the myogenic properties of smooth muscle described in the previous chapter. However, the wall of the gastrointestinal tract contains an extensive network of ganglia and nerve fibres (the intramural or intrinsic plexus) which function independently of the autonomic nervous system and contributes to the contractile activity seen *in vitro*. The myogenic properties can only be seen when conduction in the intramural nerves is blocked chemically by treating with tetrodotoxin or physically by separating the muscle from the ganglia.

When the intramural nerves are intact and functioning the segments have a far greater repertoire of movements. The contractions can be stationary as during rhythmic segmentation (see Chapter 7) and provide movements which serve to mix ingested material with digestive enzymes and bring absorbable material into contact with the mucosal surface. Peristaltic contractions propagate and provide propulsion of luminal contents. The 'peristaltic reflex' evoked by radial stretch of the intestinal wall is character-ized by an aborally directed wave of contraction arising behind the distend-ing bolus and preceded by active relaxation of the circular muscle in front of the bolus to facilitate its aboral progression. These two features of the peristaltic reflex, ascending excitation and descending inhibition, were described by Bayliss and Starling (1899) as the 'law of the intestine' because they considered them fundamental to intestinal propulsion. Coordinated contractile activity, therefore, involves both inhibitory and excitatory ner-vous mechanisms. The intramural ganglia have the additional task of coordinating the contractions of the longitudinal and circular muscle layers. Although contractions of the circular muscle produce the main force generated by the gut wall, contractions of the circular and longitudinal layer are reciprocally controlled so that each does not oppose the movements of the other.

In the absence of any external influences intramural ganglia provide the basic neural circuitry that governs the different patterns of contractile activity seen in the intact animal. The overall effect of this circuitry is best visualized by observing the effect of its removal. Tetrodotoxin has opposite effects on the two muscle layers of intestinal segments. Longitudinal muscle strips lose their contractile activity (see Bolton, 1979) while circular muscle contracts more regularly in phase with each slow wave (Wood, 1972). The longitudinal muscle layer must therefore receive a predominantly excitatory innervation while the circular muscle is tonically suppressed by its intramural nervous innervation. Further evidence for tonic inhibition of circular muscle are seen in pathological conditions where the intramural ganglia is absent. Achalasia of the oesophagus and Hirschsprung's disease are associated with spasm of the circular muscle causing an obstruction to the passage of digesta. The intramural ganglia, therefore, constantly suppress myogenic circular muscle contractions.

The ability of the intramural nerves to coordinate motility independently of the extrinsic autonomic supply led Langley in 1921 to coin the term 'enteric nervous system'. The intramural nerve ganglia can, therefore, be considered as independent of the parasympathetic and sympathetic divisions of the autonomic nervous system, although they receive connections from both and indeed the cell bodies of postganglionic parasympathetic neurones are contained within these ganglia. However, to consider the enteric nervous system as simply the relay station in the parasympathetic pathway to the gut is understating its extensiveness and complexity. In order to function as an autonomous nervous system the intramural ganglia contains essentially the same elements as the central nervous system. Sensory neurones monitoring muscle and possibly mucosal activity reflexly modify the motor output to muscle and glands. However, as in the CNS, the majority of neurones in the enteric system are neither sensory nor motor and constitute a large interneuronal pool providing the integrative ability of the intramural nerve net which allows the assimilation of information and a whole range of appropriate responses. It is no overestimate of the complexity of the system that led Wood (1981) to describe it as 'the smartest part of the gut'.

STRUCTURE OF THE INTRAMURAL GANGLIA

Intramural ganglia are found in two nerve plexuses within the gut wall (see Figure 1.1). The myenteric or Auerbach's plexus runs between the

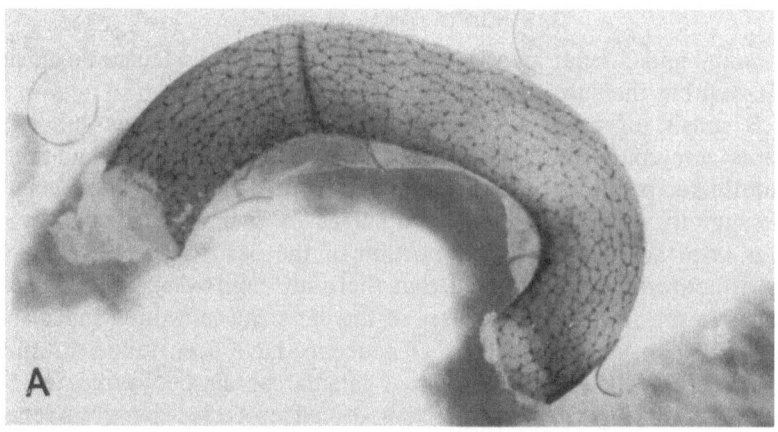

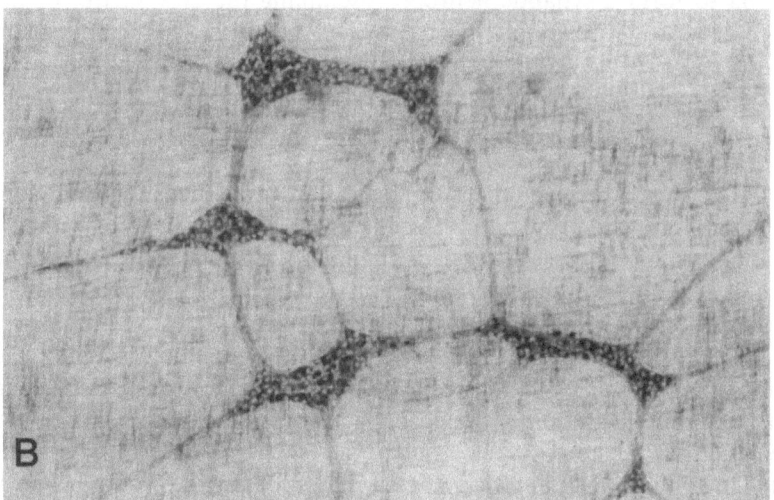

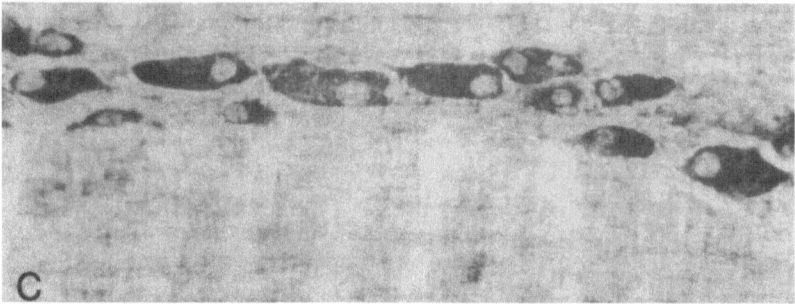

Figure 2.1 A   An intestinal loop from a chick, histochemically stained *in toto*. The myenteric plexus with its ganglia and connecting meshes is visible in the otherwise unstained wall. (From *Structure of the autonomic nervous system* by G. Gabella, 1976, with kind permission of the author and publisher, Chapman and Hall.) **B:** myenteric plexus of guinea-pig rectum stained *in toto* with a histochemical method for DPN diaphorase. Magnification 80×. The stretch preparation includes the longitudinal muscle layer which appears in the background. Three large ganglia are packed with neurones and are linked by connecting strands. **C:** nerve ganglion cells of the myenteric plexus stained as above. Magnification 480× (From Gabella, 1981, with kind permission of the author and publisher, Raven Press)

longitudinal and circular muscle, and the submucosal or Meissner's plexus is found within the submucosal layer.

Each consist of ganglia, composed of groups of neurones and glial elements, interconnected by bundles of nerve fibres (Figure 2.1) and takes on a meshlike appearance which runs uninterrupted along the whole length of the smooth muscle gut from oesophagus to anal sphincter and even extends into the striated muscle portion of the oesophagus. A detailed count of neurones has estimated that there are approximately 6 million neurones in the intramural plexuses of the cat small intestine (Sauer and Rumble, 1946). A similar density of neurones have been found in other species (see Gabella, 1981). Individual ganglia contain between 5 and 50 neurones of varying sizes and patterns of cell processes densely packed with glia to form a synaptic neuropil resembling the grey matter of the CNS. Individual neurones have been classified on the basis of their morphology into cells with several short processes and one long process (Dogiel type I) and cells with smooth surfaces and several long processes (Dogiel type II) (Figure 2.2). A third class (Dogiel type III) has both long and short processes.

Nerve fibres run between the two plexuses and interchange information, while other branches run into adjacent layers making contact with the muscle layers, blood vessels, secretory and absorptive cells, and endocrine cells. It is a fallacy, therefore, to consider that the myenteric plexus controls motor functions while the submucosal plexus controls secretion and absorption; however, in the oesophagus, where secretory function is minor, the submucosal plexus is less extensive. The myenteric plexus is also sparse in the striated muscle section of the oesophagus but why there should be any there at all is a mystery.

The analogy between enteric and central nervous system continues with the suggestion of a blood–ganglia barrier similar to the blood–brain barrier. A basal lamina surrounds individual ganglia and there are no fenestrations in adjacent capillaries. However, if a barrier does exist it is readily penetrated by the many drugs used by pharmacologists to investigate the enteric nervous system.

ELECTROPHYSIOLOGY OF INTRAMURAL PLEXUSES

Methodology

The best way of understanding the way the enteric nervous system controls gastrointestinal function is by applying similar techniques to those used to study the central nervous control of other systems – for example, voluntary movement. In this type of study the characteristics of neuronal discharge are related to the morphology of the various cell types and their interconnec-

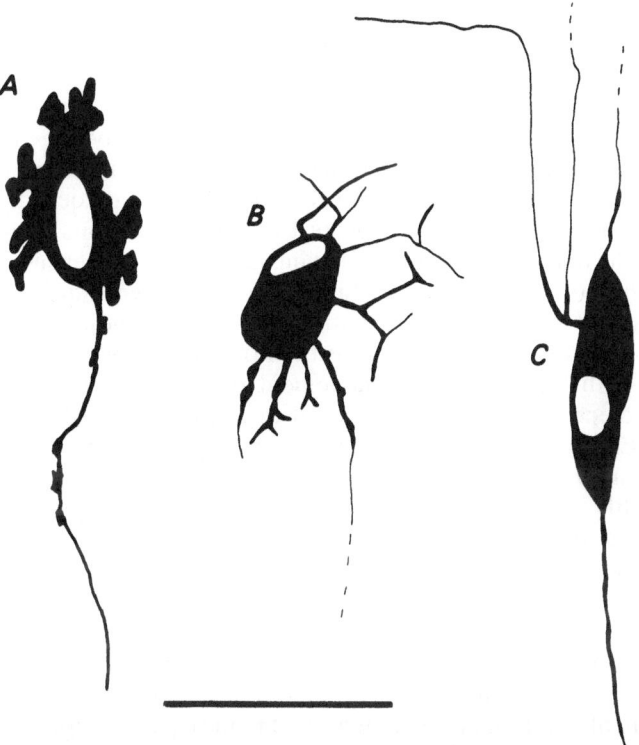

Figure 2.2 Scale drawings of myenteric neurones stained by intracellular injection of Lucifer Yellow. The cells are classified on the basis of morphology into Dogiel Type I cells (A and B) and a Dogiel Type II cell (C). Bar 50 μm (From Bornstein *et al.*, 1984, with kind permission of the authors and editor of J. Physiol. (London))

tions with other identifiable structures in the system. However, there are several difficulties associated with this approach to the enteric nervous system, first because of its diffuse structure (see Figure 2.1), and second because of its relative inaccessibility, being interspersed between the different layers that constitute the gut wall. It is important, therefore, to be able to visualize the ganglia in order to gain access with recording electrodes by removing both overlying and underlying layers of tissue. This necessitates an *in vitro* approach because disrupting the layers would also disrupt the vasculature and the resulting blood loss would obliterate the field of vision. Several methods have been employed which leave the myenteric plexus attached to either the longitudinal or the circular muscle layer. The advantage of the latter is that the submucosal plexus is still connected, but being much thicker requires a vital stain like methylene blue to enable microscopic visualization. If the plexus is left attached to the longitudinal muscle layer, which is much thinner, it allows transmitted light and therefore visualization without staining, but unfortunately disrupts the connection with the submucosal plexus. The latter can also be studied in isolation by stripping away both from above and below to leave the plexus attached to the circular muscle.

Having gained access to the ganglia, two techniques can be used to examine the properties of individual neurones. Relatively large microelectrodes can be positioned on the surface of the ganglia and neural discharge recorded extracellularly. Alternatively, much finer microelectrodes can impale individual cell soma and record intracellular events. Intracellular techniques have the advantage of allowing membrane properties of individual neurones to be examined, while extracellular techniques are easier technically and allow temporal relationships between adjacent cells to be studied in circumstances when more than one unit is detected simultaneously. In both types of study, movement of the ganglia relative to the recording electrode must be minimized to keep the recording conditions constant. Extracellular and intracellular techniques can be used to investigate spontaneous and evoked neural activity. Pharmacological treatments which modify this activity will provide insight into interconnections and neuronal circuitry.

More sophisticated techniques can be used in association with intracellular recordings of neurone activity. In addition to current injection from which the application of Ohm's law allows the cell's input resistance to be calculated, the injection of intracellular dyes allows the morphology of the cell to be correlated with its electrophysiological properties. The application of immunohistochemical techniques (see Chapter 4) further help clarify the functional significance of the various types of neurone in the enteric nervous system.

From this brief outline of the methods employed in the electrophysiological study of intramural ganglia one can appreciate the considerable technical difficulties that need to be overcome. It is for this reason that relatively few research groups have employed this approach. The guinea-pig small intestine has been used mainly in this type of study because the gut wall layers separate easily and facilitate exposure of the ganglia. However, the guinea-pig intestine shows less myogenic activity than most mammalian species, including man, and caution must be exercised when extrapolating observations on this species to others. There are, however, similarities between neural discharge recorded extracellularly in the guinea-pig and those recorded from the dog, cat and rabbit. Yet even in the guinea-pig extracellular and intracellular recordings of neuronal activity do not always correlate and, while not discrediting the conclusions of each, make the functional significance more difficult to evaluate. Since extracellular studies have led to an elegant hypothesis for the way intestinal motility is controlled, I will describe the results of these observations first.

Extracellular studies

Three distinct categories of neuronal activity have been identified in both the myenteric and submucosal plexus using extracellular recording electrodes. Of these the most interesting and probably the most controversial are the neurones which spontaneously generate (in the absence of any intentional stimulus) periodic bursts of action potentials separated by silent interburst intervals.

Burst-type neurones

Two separate populations of burst-type neurones have been described. The first, steady bursters, generate spontaneous bursts of action potentials

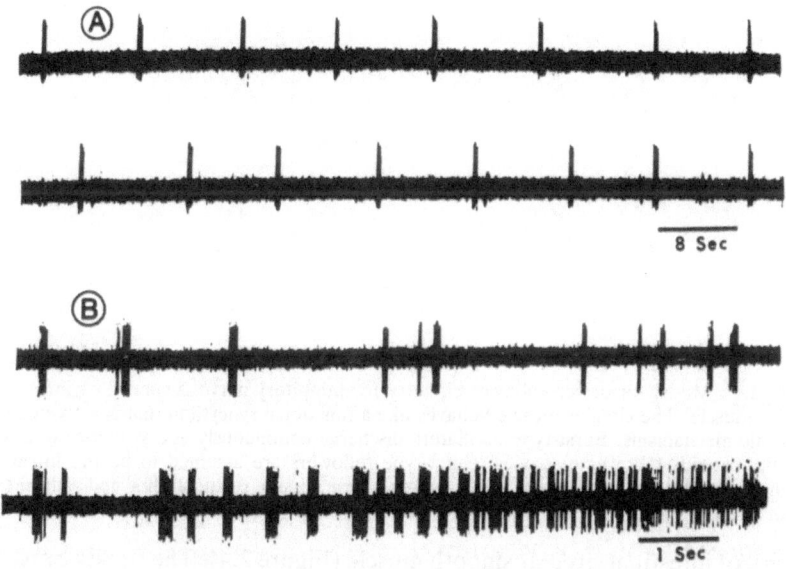

Figure 2.3 Discharge pattern of two neurones recorded extracellularly from the myenteric plexus. A: example of a steady-burst-type neurone recorded from the cat jejunum. B: example of an erratic-burst-type neurone recorded from guinea-pig jejunum (From Wood, 1975, with kind permission of the author and editor of Physiol. Rev.)

at remarkably constant intervals (Figure 2.3a). This discharge pattern continues unchanged for many hours and cannot be altered by pharmacological agents or by increasing the concentration of extracellular magnesium ions. The latter compete with calcium ions which must enter synaptic terminals prior to the release of its transmitter, and this indicates that the activity in steady burst-type cells does not depend on a synaptic input. The second type of burst-type neurones are referred to as erratic bursters because the discharge pattern is characterized by irregular interburst intervals with occasional periods of continuous discharge (see Figure 2.3b). Unlike steady bursters, these neurones depend upon a cholinergic synaptic input for their activity.

With extracellular recordings it is possible on occasions to record simultaneously from several neurones. When this occurs, temporal relationships between individual burst-type neurones can be established. Some neurones have synchronous activity suggesting that they have a common synaptic input, while other neurones have temporally coupled patterns of activity indicating that the discharge of one is driving that of another. These observations led Wood (1975) to suggest a model for the tonic inhibitory

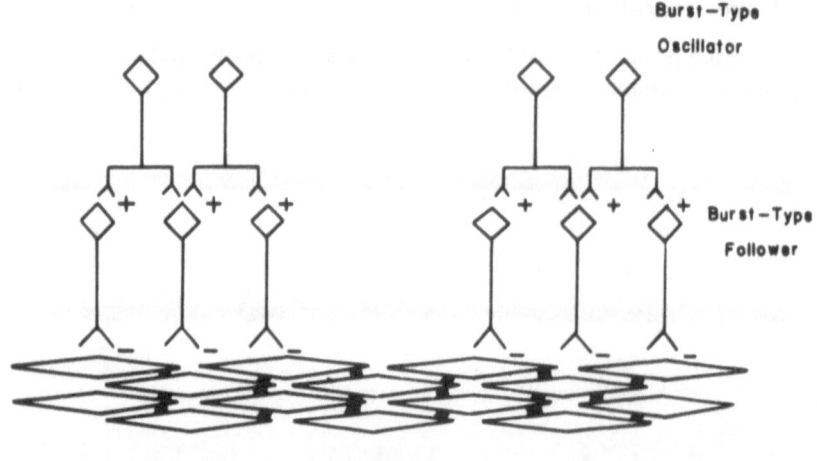

Figure 2.4 Model for driver–follower circuitry for inhibitory nervous control of intestinal circular muscle. The circular muscle behaves like a functional syncytium that is activated by myogenic mechanisms. Burst-type oscillators discharge continuously and synaptically drive non-spontaneous follower neurones. Burst-type followers are assumed to be the intrinsic inhibitory neurones (From Wood, 1981, with kind permission of the author and publisher, Raven Press)

control of intestinal circular smooth muscle (Figure 2.4). The steady burster is an endogenous oscillator which drives the erratic burster, which in turn releases an inhibitory transmitter onto the circular muscle layer. This hypothetical driver–follower circuitry would account for the continuous inhibition of circular muscle revealed when the intramural nerves are blocked. Additional synaptic inputs to the erratic 'follower' cells would provide a means of modifying the level of circular muscle inhibition by either increasing or decreasing the release of the inhibitory transmitter. The chemical nature of this transmitter is discussed in Chapter 4.

Mechanoreceptors

Sensory receptors are an essential part of any autonomous system and three types of neurone have been described as having receptor characteristics (Figure 2.5). Two of these behave as first-order sensory neurones with either rapidly or slowly adapting responses to maintained stimulation. The third type of neurone, called 'tonic-type', responds to transient stimulation

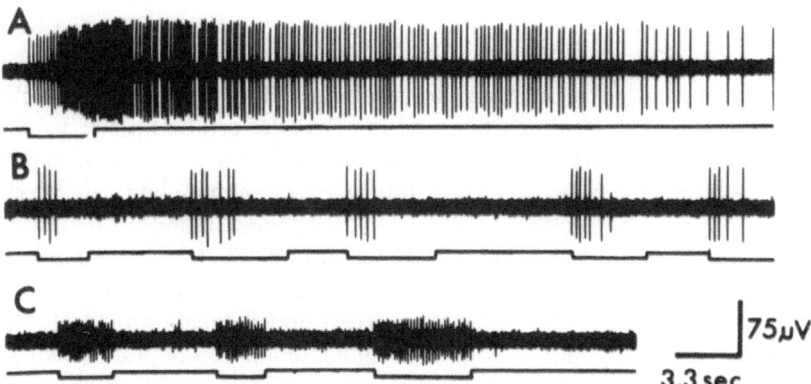

Figure 2.5 Examples of the types of mechanosensitive neurones that are detected by extracellular recording electrodes. **A:** Tonic-type mechanoreceptive neurone in myenteric plexus of cat small intestine. The unit was activated by transient mechanical deformation of the ganglionic surface (downward deflection of bottom trace) and continued to discharge long after removal of the stimulus. **B:** Rapidly adapting mechanoreceptor in myenteric plexus of cat small intestine. This unit discharged only at the onset of mechanical distortion of the ganglia. **C:** Slowly adapting mechanoreceptor in myenteric plexus of dog small intestine. This unit discharged throughout mechanical distortion (From Wood, 1981, with kind permission of the author and publisher, Raven Press)

but continues to discharge action potentials for 10–40 s after the stimulus has been removed. For this reason these are not considered as first-order sensory neurones but interneurones which are activated directly or indirectly by either the slowly or rapidly adapting mechanoreceptors.

The stimulus for receptor activation is distortion of the ganglia surface by advancing the tip of the recording electrode slightly or indenting with a glass probe. The receptive fields of these neurones, therefore, are quite distinct from sensory fibres in the parasympathetic and sympathetic nerves and, if the analogy between the enteric and central nervous systems is valid, it is equivalent to having sensory endings within the brain itself. Sensory fibres in the autonomic nervous system are of both rapidly and slowly adapting types and although these have not been identified morphologically (see Chapter 3) they are presumed from their discharge characteristics to be located in either the mucosa, muscle or serosal attachments. Any neurone wll discharge a train of action potentials when damaged (injury potentials) and this is one argument against these ganglionic neurones representing true receptors. However, one must bear in mind the unique position of enteric neurones being directly exposed to the mechanical movements that they control. Since not all ganglion cells respond in this way one might argue for a specific mechanoreceptive function rather than a non-specific response to distortion.

The mechanoreceptive neurones have been incorporated into the driver–follower hypothesis for the control of the circular muscle layer.

25

Receptor activation is proposed to be reinforced by prolonged discharge in the tonic-type neurones which synapse on the erratic burster. Inhibition of the erratic burster would lead to contraction by releasing the muscle from its inhibitory restraint while excitation of the erratic burster would release more inhibitory transmitter and cause relaxation. The two major motor patterns seen in the small intestine are segmentation and peristalsis. A segmentatory contraction would occur if the tonic inhibitory neurones innervating a narrow region of intestine were suppressed allowing a myogenic contraction to develop. The degree of suppression would regulate the force of contraction. To prevent the contraction propagating through the smooth muscle syncytium to adjacent regions, enhanced neural discharge would be required to hyperpolarize these areas. The motor programme for segmentation is, therefore, proposed to involve reciprocal inhibition and disinhibition of adjacent segments of intestine.

Peristaltic contractions generally propagate in the aboral direction but under special circumstances, for example during vomiting or when the intestine develops a blockage, can spread in the opposite direction. One can envisage peristalsis, in either direction, as occurring when regions of circular muscle are disinhibited in sequence allowing myogenic contractions to propagate along a length of intestine.

Single spike neurones

The last group of neurones identified on the basis of their spontaneous discharge characteristics are the single spike neurones. As the name implies these neurones show continuous low frequency randomly separated action potentials. This discharge depends partly on a synaptic input since it is altered but never blocked by a high concentration of magnesium ions in the external medium. These cells, therefore, receive a synaptic input but are not totally dependent on it. Topical applications of acetylcholine act on nicotinic receptors to increase the frequency at which action potentials are generated. Noradrenaline acts on alpha receptors to produce the opposite effect. These properties are reminiscent of postganglionic parasympathetic fibres (see Chapter 3) and this may be one possible role for this type of neurone.

Most postganglionic parasympathetic neurones release acetylcholine as their transmitter substance. Since, from the driver–follower hypothesis the major innervation to the circular muscle layer is an inhibitory one, one might presume that this innervation is to the longitudinal muscle layer. The implication of this is again discussed later since in the small intestine the longitudinal muscle is believed to be the source of the slow waves which govern myogenic contractility.

Intracellular recordings

Intracellular recordings from enteric neurones, being technically more difficult, lagged a few years behind the extracellular studies but were reported independently and almost simultaneously by two research groups (Nishi and North, 1973; Hirst, Holman and Spence, 1974). Both studies revealed only two types of neurone in the guinea-pig small intestine. The first type predominated in both plexuses and were called type 1 by Nishi and North (1973) and S cells by Hirst et al. (1974), because of the presence of spontaneous membrane depolarizations indicating synaptic bombardment. The excitatory postsynaptic potentials occasionally reached threshold and generated spontaneous action potentials. During the intra-cellular injection of depolarizing current these cells discharged action potentials repeatedly (Figure 2.6). The excitatory postsynaptic potentials were mimicked by iontophoresis of acetylcholine and blocked by nicotinic cholinergic blockade.

The second type of neurone, detected more readily in the myenteric than submucosal plexus, had very different properties from the S cell and was termed type 2 by Nishi and North (1973) and AH cell by Hirst et al. (1974). The AH abbreviation refers to the prolonged hyperpolarization lasting up to 30 s following the generation of an action potential (Figure 2.7). Unlike the S cells, these AH cells showed no spontaneous action potentials. Action potentials could be evoked by depolarizing current injection but only at the beginning of prolonged depolarizing pulses. The hyperpolarization therefore limits the ability of these cells to generate action potentials. Input resistance measurements demonstrate an increase in membrane conduct-ance during the afterhyperpolarization that is reversed at the equilibrium potential for potassium ions. The AH cell action potential is not blocked by tetrodotoxin and represents a novel type of nerve action potential that depends on the influx of calcium ions which triggers the potassium efflux responsible for the afterhyperpolarization. The lack of spontaneous activity in these AH cells and their unresponsiveness to iontophoretic applications of acetylcholine led to the idea that they were sensory cells. The S type neurones are considered as interneurones or motor neurones that are either excitatory or inhibitory to the smooth muscle layers.

The most obvious difference between the results of these intracellular studies and the extracellular studies described earlier is the lack of any inherent pacemaker activity (burst-type cells). In fact, spontaneous action potentials are a relatively rare phenomenon when recording with intracellu-lar electrodes and when these do occur they represent synaptic input to a cell process invading the cell body, and not spontaneous generation of action potentials. A critical explanation of these differences suggests that the various types of neurone recorded with extracellular electrodes rep-resent differing degrees of mechanical deformation brought about by the large extracellular electrodes (North, 1982). Intracellular electrodes, hav-ing much finer tips, cause less damage. Mechanical damage to AH cells could conceivably generate a cyclical pattern of discharge due to the

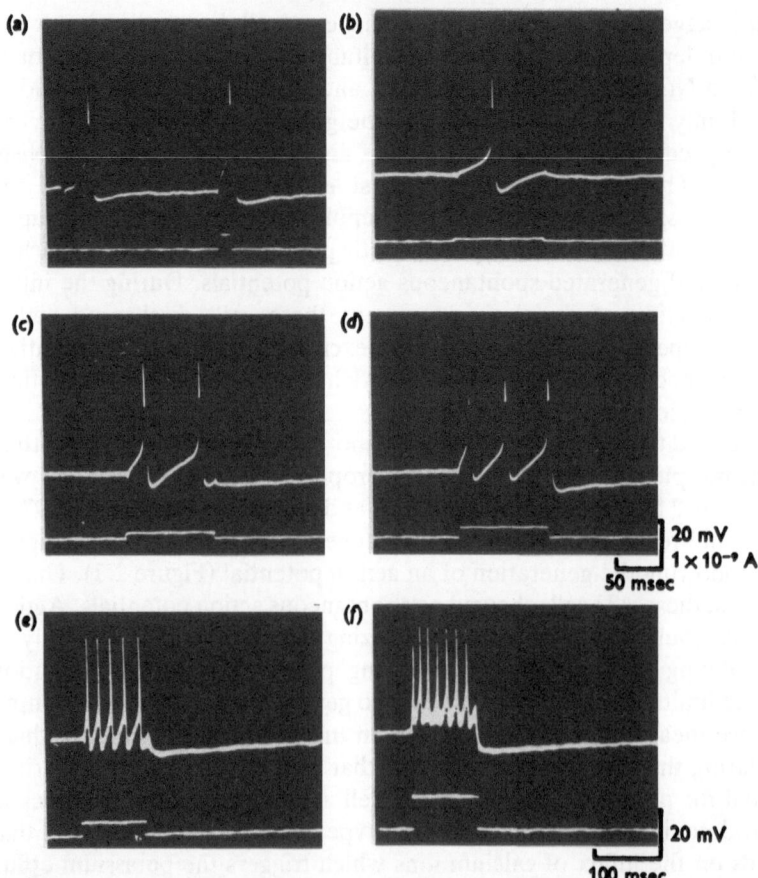

Figure 2.6 Action potentials generated by a S cell in the myenteric plexus of guinea-pig duodenum. In (a) the first action potential was initiated by transmural electrical stimulation, the second was initiated by passing a brief current pulse through the recording electrode. The effect of increasing the intensity of current is shown in **b–f**. The upper trace records the intracellular potential while the lower trace shows the duration and intensity of the current pulse (From Hirst *et al.*, 1974, with kind permission of the author and editor of J. Physiol. (London))

afterhyperpolarization limiting the cells firing ability. Similarly, rapidly adapting mechanoreceptors may represent transient distortion of an AH cell while slowly adapting reponses might be expected when a S-type cell is deformed. Wood and Mayer (1978) in their intracellular studies, also failed to detect an endogenous oscillator but suggests that they may go undetected if the cells are too small to impale with microelectrodes. The argument is at present unresolved and further details can be obtained from recent reviews by North (1982) and Wood (1981).

The single spike cells recorded extracellularly are suggested to be the least damaged and this reflects their similarity to S-type cells. The sugges-

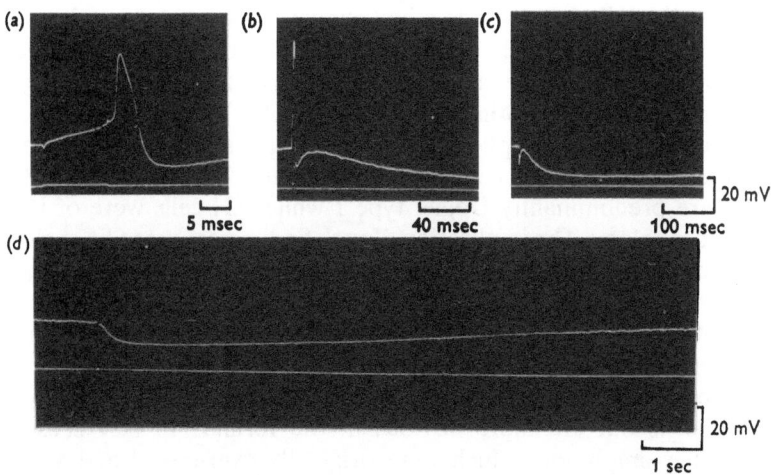

Figure 2.7 Action potentials generated by an AH cell in the myenteric plexus of guinea-pig duodenum during the passage of current through the microelectrode. The responses of four cells are illustrated at different recording speeds. In **d** the action potential is not obvious but the long period of after hyperpolarization is clearly seen (From Hirst *et al.*, 1974, with kind permission of the author and editor of J. Physiol. (London))

tion that single spike cells represent postganglionic parasympathetic neurones may be borne out by a recent observation of ganglionic transmission in the opossum stomach (King and Szurszewski, 1984). Small ganglia can be identified within the gut wall in close proximitiy to branches of the vagal supply (parafascicular ganglia). Intracellular recordings from these ganglia revealed only S-type cells which received synaptic inputs from a number of vagal fascicles.

Synaptic potentials

Individual ganglia receive synaptic connections from adjacent ganglia via the bundles of interconnecting fibres. Electrical stimulation of these bundles or neighbouring ganglia will therefore evoke responses in ganglia which can be detected using either intracellular or extracellular recording techniques. Evoked responses can be detected in the longitudinal direction up to 15mm from the point of stimulation, while in the circular direction the spread of excitation is very much less (Yokoyama, 1971). The orientation of synaptic connections therefore favours transmission in the longitudinal direction. That these evoked responses did indeed depend on synaptic connections was demonstrated by their sensitivity to pharmacological agents which interfered with nicotinic cholinoreceptors. An observation which also explains why such drugs block the peristaltic reflex.

The morphology of individual cells does not necessarily support the electrophysiological data. In the studies of Hodgkiss and Lees (1980) individual neurones were injected with Procian yellow after first classifying the cells as of AH or S type. The majority of long processes occurred not in the longitudinal direction as one might expect but in a circular orientation. However, the longitudinally directed processes that were identified occurred predominantly in the aboral direction indicating a preference for descending pathways. Another study using Lucifer Yellow as an intracellular marker compared morphology with electrophysiology and demonstrated a relationship between cell shape and function (Bornstein *et al.*, 1984). S cells were predominantly Dogiel type I while AH cells were of Dogiel type II morphology. The implication of such findings are yet to be evaluated but support the original suggestion that S cells are either interneurones or motor neurones.

Intracellular recordings of synaptic transmission from adjacent ganglia reveal both excitatory and inhibitory synaptic potentials. Fast excitatory postsynaptic potentials (epsp) of short duration (20–60 ms) occur in both S and AH cells but are more obvious in the former. In AH cells epsp have smaller amplitudes which were originally overlooked and are only discriminated from background noise by signal averaging techniques. The small amplitude of these potentials probably reflect synaptic input to a region of the cell well away from the recording site within the cell body. The epsp in both cell types are mediated through acetylcholine acting on nicotinic receptors.

Slow epsp can be elicited in AH cells following repetitive electrical stimulation of the fibre bundles innervating a particular ganglion. The duration of these are over 1000 times longer than the fast epsp and have a remarkable transforming effect on the properties of the AH cell (Wood, 1981). It is converted from the relatively unresponsive cell described above to one which discharges a train of action potentials that persist for several seconds following the removal of the stimulus (Figure 2.8). The postspike hyperpolarization is greatly reduced during the slow epsp because of a reduction in the membrane conductance to potassium ions. The consequence of this is the greatly increased excitability of these cells. The functional significance of this slow epsp relates to the similarity between this response and the response of the tonic-type mechanoreceptor to ganglionic distortion, and provides a mechanism for the production of sustained excitation or inhibition at neuronal or neuromuscular junctions.

Inhibitory postsynaptic potentials (ipsp) are a rare feature of synaptic activity in the enteric nervous system, especially in the myenteric plexus. They appear to depend upon release of a catecholamine transmitter of intrinsic nervous origin and may be involved in delaying the onset of excitatory transmission in the submucosal plexus (see below, p. 32). Inhibitory events would increase the integrative capacity of the enteric nervous system and would be an essential component of the peristaltic reflex if this occurs through disinhibition of the circular muscle layer.

Nerve pathways in the enteric nervous system

The studies described so far suffer from the same inherent problem of

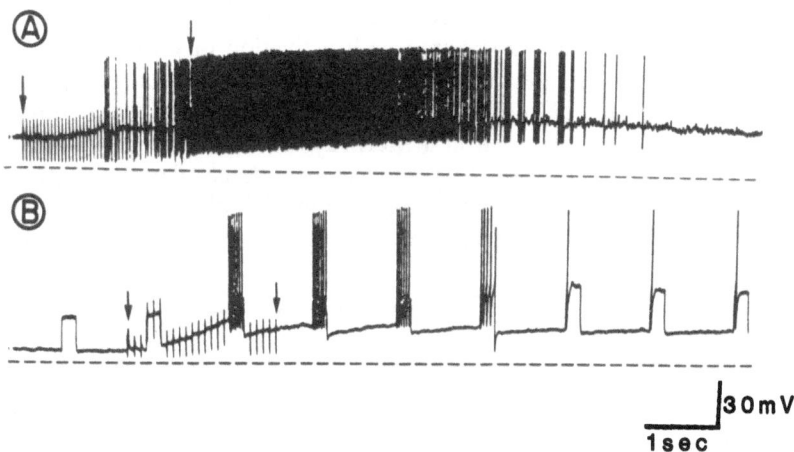

Figure 2.8 Slow synaptic excitation in an AH cell recorded from the myenteric plexus of guinea-pig small intestine. A: Slow epsp and spike discharge elicited by electrical stimulation of the interganglionic fibre tract (arrows indicate duration of stimulus pulse train). B: Electrical stimulation of the fibre tract caused an increase in excitability as indicated by spike discharge throughout constant current depolarizing pulses (From Wood, 1981, with kind permission of the author and publisher, Raven Press)

requiring isolation of strips of intestine. These preparations therefore lack continuity of the gut and its associated plexus. Hirst and McKirdy (1974) used a slightly different technique to get round this problem. They recorded intracellularly from myenteric neurones on the surface of a flap of stripped longitudinal muscle which was still connected to an intact 5 cm loop of small intestine. Flaps could be made from either end of the intestinal segments and essential differences were detected between orally and aborally directed flaps. Atropine was required in the bathing medium to prevent acetylcholine, liberated from nerve terminals, inducing contractions that would make impaling the myenteric cells difficult.

S type myenteric cells in anally directed flaps showed spontaneous epsp which on occasions reached threshold for the generation of action potentials. These cells therefore received continuous synaptic bombardment from an ascending source that was enhanced by distension of the loop or transmural electrical stimulation of the intestinal segment. The synaptic potential evoked by such procedures occurred after a variable latency from the application of the stimulus to the start of the response. Analysis of this latency indicated that myenteric neurones could be separated into two populations of neurones. One group of neurones had a short latency response of between 0.2 and 1.2 s while the other group had a latency of between 2 and 11 s. Orally directed flaps showed no spontaneous activity and very few cells responded to transmural stimulation. Therefore, descending pathways predominate, of which two can be separated on the basis of

31

latency. No AH cells showed any evidence of a synaptic input, be it fast or slow and no ipsp were recorded in this preparation.

The mechanical effects associated with activation of these descending pathways were investigated by making intracellular recordings from the muscle cells of both longitudinal and circular muscle during reflex stimulation as above (Hirst, Holman and McKirdy, 1975). When atropine was present in the bathing medium no responses were detected in the longitudinal layer. However, transient hyperpolarizations (inhibitory junction potentials) were detected in the circular muscle after a latency corresponding to

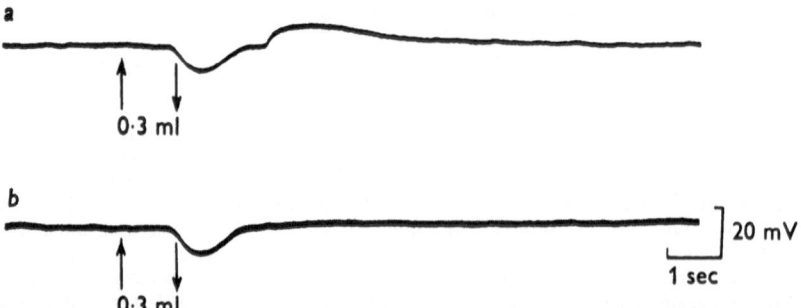

Figure 2.9 Intracellular recordings from circular muscle layer of guinea-pig small intestine showing the sequence of changes in membrane potential evoked by a brief distension of an orally situated segment of intestine. **a** was recorded in drug free solution while **b** was the response 8 min after changing to a solution containing atropine $(2 \times 10^{-7} \text{g ml}^{-1})$ (From Hirst *et al.*, 1975, with kind permission of the author and editor of J. Physiol.(London))

activation of the short latency pathway (Figure 2.9). Sensory neurones in the muscle or myenteric plexus (the reflex continues after removal of the mucosal layers) are therefore activated by distension which excites a descending chain of neurones and bring about inhibition of the circular muscle. This, therefore, represents the descending inhibitory pathway which is an essential component of Bayliss and Starling's 'Law of the Intestine'.

In the absence of atropine, distension caused a ring of contraction to develop in the circular muscle above the site of the distension which then propagated aborally. Movement resulting from these contractions generally dislodged the recording electrodes, but where recordings remained stable a longer latency depolarization (excitatory junction potential) was seen in both muscle layers. In the circular muscle this depolarization was preceded by the shorter latency hyperpolarization (see Figure 2.9). The excitatory response was abolished by removing the submucosal plexus and this is thought to be the site for the delay in synaptic transmission of the descending excitation.

These two pathways are shown schematically in Figure 2.10. During the peristaltic reflex there is a phase of descending inhibition which makes the gut receptive for the phase of descending excitation that follows. The latter provides the propulsive force that moves intestinal contents along the gut.

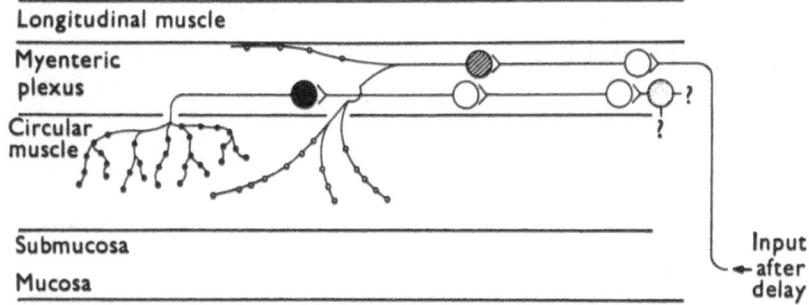

Figure 2.10 Schematic representation of the two descending nerve pathways. The lower pathway represents the descending inhibitory pathway. An AH cell (cell body stippled) is in some way activated by distension; its efferent process impinges on a chain of cholinergic interneurones (open circles) which in turn activate an inhibitory neurone (large filled circle). Inhibitory fibres, runing in an anal direction, terminate on the circular muscle. The upper pathway represents the descending excitatory pathway. Input to this pathway occurs after a delay that involves transmission through the submucous plexus. Both interneurones (open circles) and excitatory neurones (hatched circles) are activated (From Hirst *et al.*, 1975, with kind permission of the author and editor of J. Physiol.(London))

MODEL FOR PERISTALSIS

How can the data from these different, and sometimes conflicting, electro-physiological studies be reconciled into a unifying hypothesis for the enteric nervous control of intestinal motility? Figure 2.11 shows one such attempt although several points need qualifying. Firstly, atropine, the muscarinic cholinoreceptor antagonist, blocks the excitatory junction potential and hence contraction of the circular muscle evoked by distension or transmural electrical stimulation of intestinal segments. According to the 'driver–follower' hypothesis contractions are achieved by disinhibition of a tonically active inhibitory innervation. In the scheme shown in Figure 2.11 contraction of the circular muscle layer is proposed to arise by a combination of cholinergic excitation and disinhibition of the release of an inhibitory transmitter suggested in this model to be ATP (see Chapter 4).

An alternative way of reconciling these conflicting observations involves contractions of the longitudinal muscle layer which occur out of phase with circular muscle contractions. The longitudinal muscle receives a predominantly excitatory innervation and being the source of the myogenic slow wave could trigger circular muscle contractions to follow should the slow waves reach threshold because of the release of acetylcholine. Electrotonic current spread from the longitudinal muscle to the circular coat could generate sequential rings of contraction that consequently result in the propagation of a wave of contraction passing along a segment of intestine. There is some anatomical evidence for coupling between the two muscle layers. The exchange of smooth muscle cells between adjacent muscle layers has been proposed while another site of coupling may be the

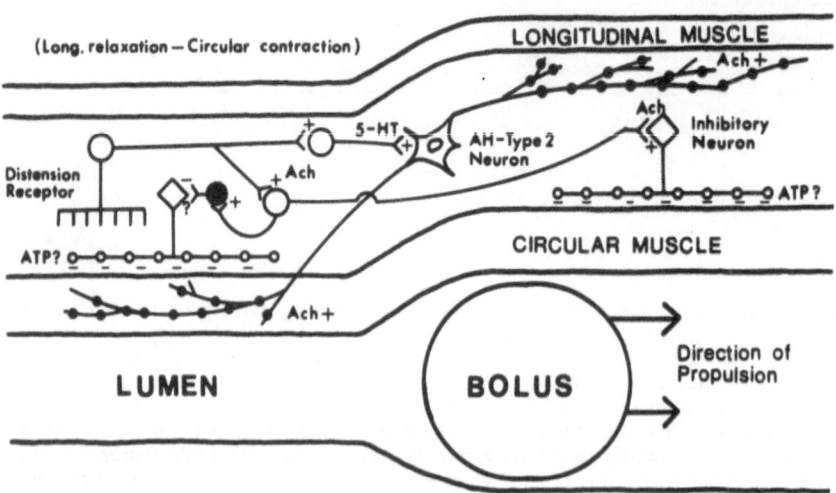

Figure 2.11 Schematic neural circuitry for control of the intestinal muscle layers during peristaltic propulsion of an intraluminal bolus. Putative neurotransmitters are given; (+) indicates an excitatory synapse; (−) an inhibitory synapse (From Wood, 1981, with kind permission of the author and publisher, Raven Press)

interstitial cells of Cajal which make nexus connections with smooth muscle cells and may bridge the gap across the myenteric plexus (Gabella, 1981). However, evidence exists against coupling of the muscle layers. Contractions can occur in the circular muscle independently of contractions in the longitudinal muscle. Atropine, for example, blocks longitudinal contractions at a lower dose than that required to prevent contractions in the circular layer. Contractions of the longitudinal layer are not, therefore, a prerequisite for circular mucle contractions.

One piece of evidence lacking from the scheme in Figure 2.11 is an electrophysiological basis for the ascending excitatory pathway that generates the contraction orad to the distending bolus. Evidence for such a pathway stems from observations of mechanical events associated with peristalsis. In the colon this ascending excitation extends measurably for some way (Costa and Furness, 1976). However, in the small intestine this orad projection is very much shorter and was not detected electrophysiologically because of the difficulty in recording so near the site of stimulation.

There is still some way to go before the complexity of the enteric nervous system is completely unravelled. However, it is evident that complex contractile activity is programmed by the intramural nerves. Extrinsic nerves and hormones regulate the motor programme so that motility in the digestive system is matched to the needs of the individual.

3
Extrinsic innervation

INTRODUCTION

The autonomic nervous system makes widespread connections with the gastrointestinal tract and electrical stimulation of the nerve bundles innervating the various gut regions have profound effects on motility. Yet removal of the extrinsic nerve supply has in most regions only a limited effect on motor activity. Only in the upper oesophagus and the external anal sphincter, where the motor function is performed by striated muscle, is there total loss of muscular contractility when the parasympathetic supply is disrupted. The rest of the gastrointestinal tract, being composed of smooth muscle with its own intrinsic nerve supply, does not show this absolute dependence on its motor innervation. Instead, denervation is followed, at worst, by a transient period of disorganized activity lasting from a few days to several weeks during which time there is a gradual return to normal activity.

It is because the effects of denervation are unspectacular that the importance of the extrinsic innervation in controlling gastrointestinal motility has been questioned. One line of argument gauges the importance of the extrinsic supply from the relative number of autonomic nerve fibres compared to the number of neurones in the intramural plexuses. The autonomic nerves innervating the gastrointestinal tract are composed of probably no more than 100000 nerve fibres of which the majority are afferent fibres carrying sensory information from the viscera to the central nervous system. The ratio of afferent to efferent fibres in the abdominal vagus nerves of the cat, for example, is about 10:1 from a total number of about 31000 fibres (Agostoni et al., 1957). Since the efferent fibres serve many digestive functions relating to secretion, absorption and blood flow the number involved in the regulation of motility is probably quite small.

However, as discussed in Chapter 2, the enteric nervous system with its millions of neurones provides the preprogrammed neural network that determines the different motor patterns seen in the various regions of the

35

gastrointestinal tract. All that is required of the extrinsic nerves, therefore, is to provide a controlling mechanism to regulate the hard-wired enteric motor programmes to the overall needs of the individual. As such the extrinsic nerves coordinate motility of the different regions of the gut which in man can be up to 7 meters apart but in animals like the pig and sheep is considerably longer. Thus, sectioning the extrinsic nerves, while not paralysing the gut, does have serious disruptive effects. These, however, are only short lived with relatively normal functioning returning long before any sign of reinnervation because of the remarkable ability of the intrinsic nervous supply to adapt to the loss of its extrinsic innervation.

In this chapter the general organization of the autonomic innervation is discussed. How this innervation affects specific regions of the gastrointestinal tract is discussed in detail in Chapters 5 to 8.

GROSS ANATOMY OF THE EXTRINSIC NERVE SUPPLY

While the separation of the autonomic nervous system into parasympathetic and sympathetic divisions on the basis of anatomical differences is still valid today, the classical view that they operate as antagonistic pathways under separate conditions of restful digestion and flight or fright is no longer tenable.

In Figures 3.1 and 3.2 the distribution of the parasympathetic and sympathetic divisions of the autonomic supply to the gastrointestinal tract are illustrated schematically. Note that these figures illustrate only the efferent side of the innervation. The distribution of sensory fibres in the parasympathetic and sympathetic nerves is equally extensive and in terms of numbers provides the largest proportion of the innervation. Afferent fibres largely follow the same route to the CNS as the efferent fibres leaving it and so can be divided broadly into parasympathetic and sympathetic afferent fibres. More important differences relate to their receptive properties and are described in detail on p. 44.

The parasympathetic supply

The parasympathetic supply to the gastrointestinal tract arises in two separate regions of the CNS. One source is the brainstem which contains the cells of origin of the vagal supply to the viscera. These are located in two nuclei, the dorsomotor vagal nucleus and the nucleus ambiguus, lying in close proximity in the medulla oblongata (Figure 3.3). The latter provide the motor innervation to the striated muscle portion of the oesophagus while the former are the preganglionic neurones proper of the parasympathetic outflow. The second source of parasympathetic efferent fibres is the posterolateral parts of the anterior columns of the sacral spinal cord

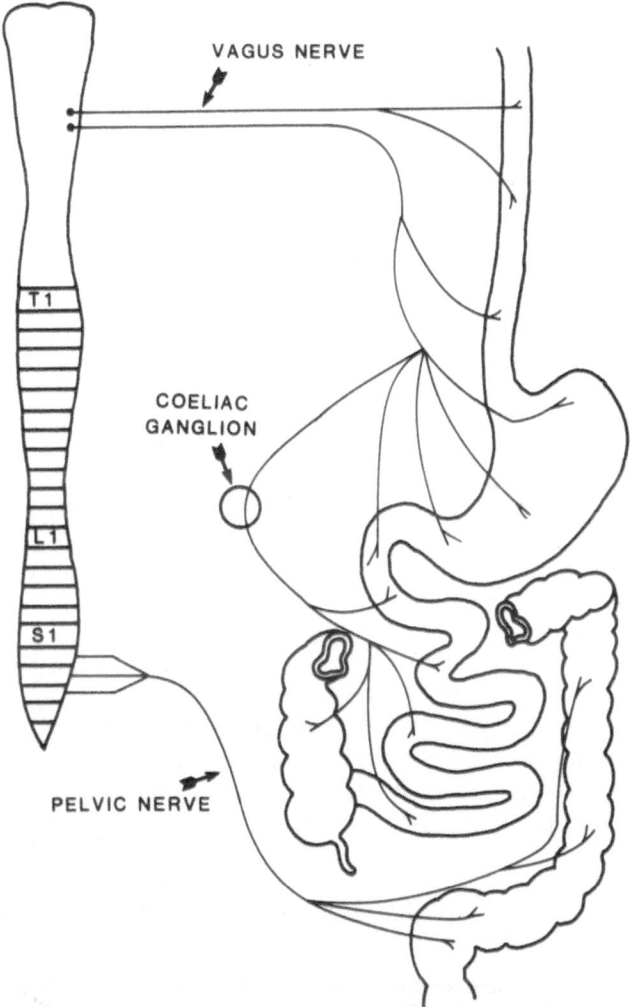

Figure 3.1 Parasympathetic innervation of the gastrointestinal tract showing only the preganglionic efferent supply; the postganglionic parasympathetic neurones (not shown) are located intramurally. (Modified from Goyal, 1978)

which is the origin of the pelvic nerves. The vagus nerves innervate the oesophagus, stomach, small intestine, proximal colon and possibly further although in these distal regions the pelvic supply from the sacral cord becomes increasingly important. The vagus nerves branch soon after entering the abdomen with major trunks supplying the stomach and liver. The nerves destined for more distal regions travel predominantly in the coeliac branch of the vagus nerves and reach the intestines via the paravascular nerve bundles which also contain the postganglionic sympathetic nerves.

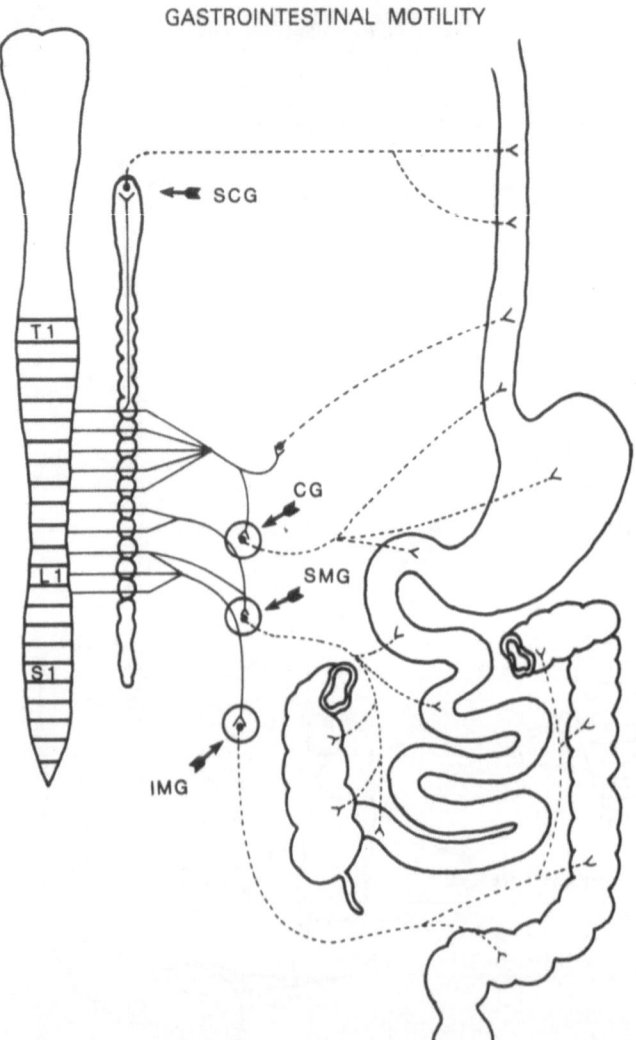

Figure 3.2 Sympathetic innervation of the gastrointestinal tract. Preganglionic neurones are represented by solid lines; postganglionic sympathetic neurones have their cell bodies in the prevertebral ganglia and are shown as broken lines. Symbols: SCG = superior cervical ganglia; CG = coeliac ganglia; SMG = superior mesenteric ganglia; IMG = inferior mesenteric ganglia (Modified from Goyal, 1978)

The vagal fibres are mainly small diameter, slowly conducting C fibres. However, the fibres innervating the upper oesophagus are myelinated and consequently conduct impulses at faster velocities. The terminations of the preganglionic parasympathetic axons are on ganglionic neurones in the intramural plexuses (not shown in Figure 3.1). The postganglionic parasympathetic neurones thus form part of the enteric nervous system and it is suggested that they provide the final common pathway to the muscle for both long reflexes via the parasympathetic nerves and short reflexes within the plexuses (Langley, 1921).

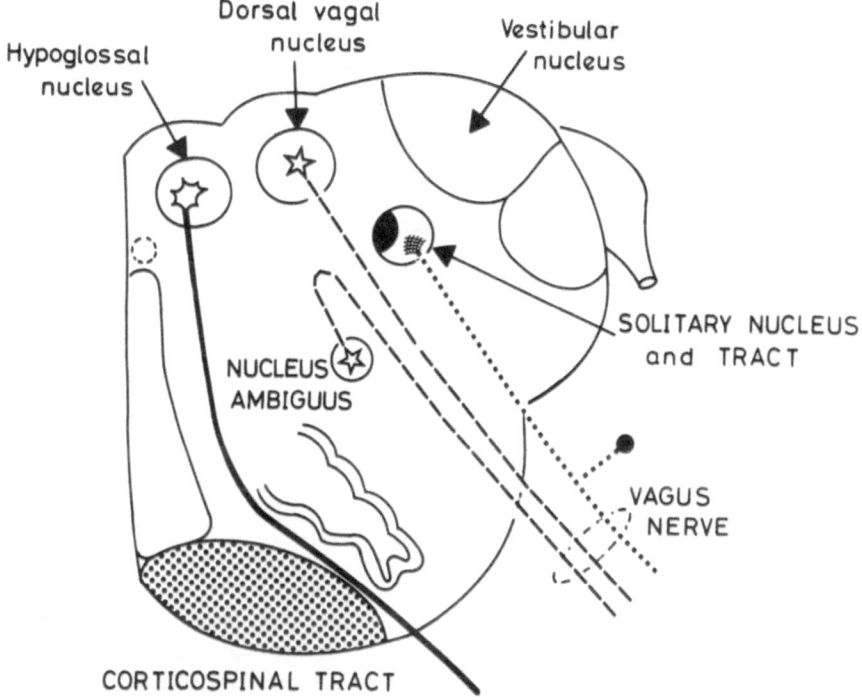

Figure 3.3 Vagal supply to the viscera. Afferent fibres with cell bodies in the jugular or nodose ganglia terminate in the nucleus of the tractus solitarius. Efferent fibres originate in the dorsal vagal nucleus and the nucleus ambiguus. The latter provides the somatic nerves innervating skeletal muscle in the upper oesophagus

Chemical transmission in the parasympathetic pathway is classically described as being mediated by acetylcholine. Nicotine prevents ganglionic transmission while the contractile response to transmitter release from postganglionic endings is blocked by atropine. After treatment with atropine, however, vagal stimulation causes relaxation of the lower oesophageal sphincter and stomach indicating that the vagus nerve is not purely excitatory but also contains an inhibitory pathway. This inhibitory response was originally attributed to the presence of sympathetic fibres in the cervical sympathetic nerves which run parallel with the vagus nerve in the neck (the so-called vagosympathetic trunk). However, the majority of these sympathetic fibres innervate the thorax with few reaching the abdomen. Subsequent use of adrenergic antagonists confirmed that this inhibitory pathway in the vagus nerve was neither cholinergic nor adrenergic, and while the nature of the transmitter remains unknown (see Chapter 4) is somewhat clumsily referred to as the non-adrenergic, non-cholinergic inhibitory pathway.

The sympathetic supply

The sympathetic preganglionic fibres arise in the intermediolateral columns of the thoracic and lumbar regions of the spinal cord, leave via the ventral roots and travel in the white rami communicans although they pass through

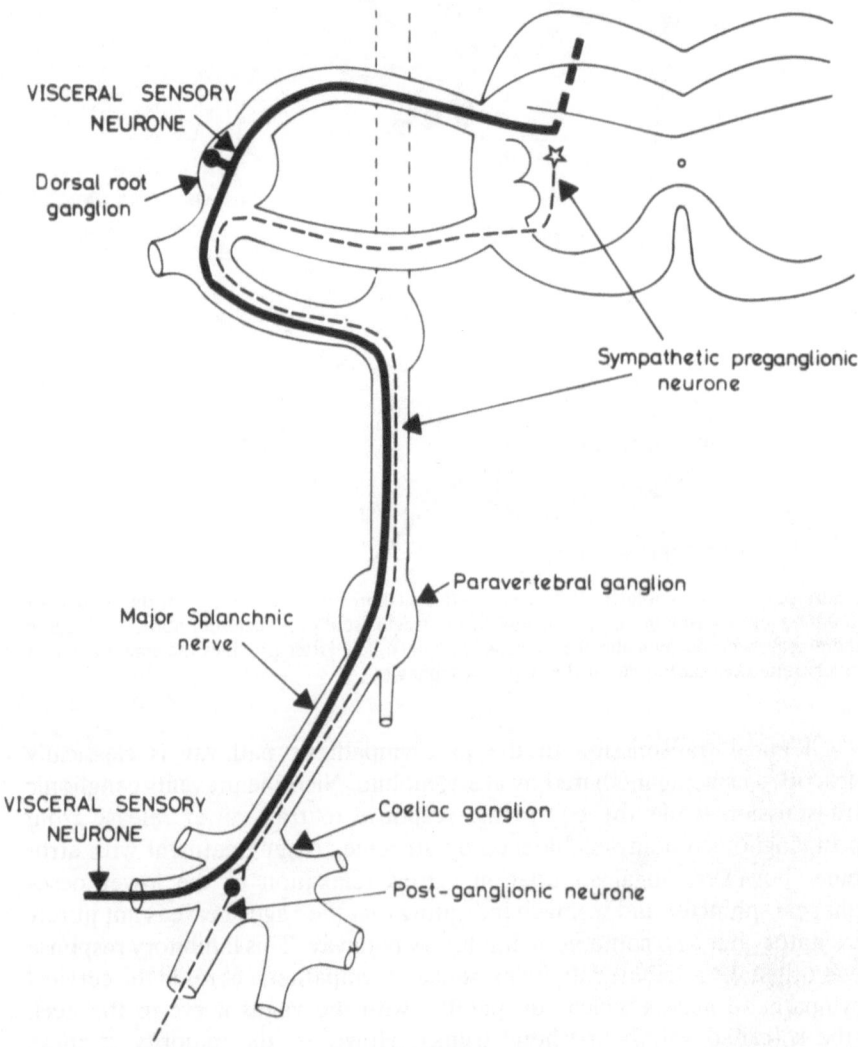

Figure 3.4 Splanchnic supply to the proximal gut. Afferent neurones have cell bodies in the dorsal root ganglia and enter the cord mainly via the dorsal roots. The preganglionic neurones pass through the sympathetic chain and terminate in the prevertebral ganglia

the sympathetic chain without making synaptic contact (Figure 3.4). They terminate on postganglionic noradrenergic neurones in the prevertebral ganglia (see Figure 3.2). Generally speaking preganglionic neurones from spinal segments T_5 to T_{12} reach the coeliac and superior mesenteric ganglia via the greater, lesser and least thoracic splanchnic nerves while the inferior mesenteric ganglia receive preganglionic inputs from T_{12} to L_3 via the lumbar splanchnic nerves. Each of the prevertebral ganglia, however, are interconnected by the intermesenteric nerves so that the interchange of nerve fibres between ganglia is considerable and make definitive statements regarding the source of preganglionic inputs impossible. Postganglionic neurones from the coeliac ganglion innervate the stomach and small intestine, the superior mesenteric ganglion supplies the distal small intestine and proximal colon while the inferior mesenteric ganglion innervates the distal colon and rectum. The bundles of postganglionic sympathetic nerves may also contain some preganglionic parasympathetic fibres from the coeliac branch of the vagus nerve (see Figure 3.1) and collectively constitute the mesenteric and colonic nerves. These are therefore mixed parasympathetic and sympathetic nerves and consist of between three and six fine nerve bundles which accompany the arterial vessels supplying the gastrointestinal tract and are hence referred to as the paravascular nerves. The postganglionic sympathetic nerves are, like the preganglionic parasympathetic nerves, small-diameter unmyelinated fibres although the preganglionic sympathetic fibres are predominantly myelinated.

The idea that the postganglionic sympathetic fibres, like the preganglionic parasympathetic fibres, innervated the intramural plexuses and not the smooth muscle directly stemmed from observation by Norberg (1964) using the Falck–Hillarp technique to stain noradrenergic terminals. The adrenergic terminals were found mainly on the surface of ganglia and not within the muscle layers and so were postulated to have a predominantly ganglionic site of action (see Figure 4.3, p. 62). A similar conclusion was reached by Jannsen and Martinson (1966) who demonstrated that, in the cat, inhibition of gastric motility by electrical stimulation of the sympathetic nerve depended upon an intact vagal supply. After vagal section the response to sympathetic stimulation was markedly reduced, but it returned if the vagus nerves were electrically stimulated. The interpretation of these data was that the sympathetic nerves acted predominantly on the vagal excitatory pathway at the level of the intramural plexus. Andrews and Lawes (1984), on the other hand, found that in the ferret the gastric response to reflex sympathetic activation was more evident after vagal section or after atropinization providing time was allowed for tone in the stomach to be re-established after each treatment. These authors propose, therefore, a direct effect of the sympathetically released noradrenaline on gastric smooth muscle. Thus the sympathetics may act at several different levels: preganglionically on the vagal excitatory pathway, on postganglionic neurones; or directly on the muscle itself. These findings are discussed further in Chapter 4.

Hierarchy of autonomic controls

Activity in the enteric nervous system is modified by synaptic inputs from both parasympathetic and sympathetic nerves. The magnitude of this extrinsic influence depends on reflex excitation or inhibition from visceral afferent fibres and from descending pathways in the CNS. The afferent fibres in the sympathetic and sacral parasympathetic nerves have their cell bodies in the dorsal root ganglion although a significant number of afferent nerve axons enter the cord via the ventral roots. The parasympathetic sensory cell bodies lie in the vagal nodose and jugular ganglia lying at the base of the skull and terminate in the brain stem in the region of the nucleus of tractus solitarius (see Figure 3.3). Other sensory fibres with cell bodies within the intramural plexuses project into the prevertebral ganglia where they can reflexly modify the sympathetic postganglionic supply.

This arrangement provides a hierarchy of neural controls (Figure 3.5). The intramural nerves provide the first level of integration allowing complex motor control in the absence of an extrinsic supply. The second level of integration occurs in the prevertebral ganglia where a peripheral reflex arc is influenced by preganglionic fibres from the spinal cord. The highest level of control is within the CNS itself. Here the outflow in the autonomic nerves is determined by reflexes whose afferent pathways reach the CNS also in autonomic nerves, and integrate with descending impulses from higher centres.

AFFERENT INNERVATION OF THE GASTROINTESTINAL TRACT

Afferent fibres greatly outnumber efferent fibres in autonomic nerves innervating the viscera and play an important role in the reflex control of the gut. Unfortunately, however, they are often ignored in general descriptions of the autonomic nervous system. This is because sensory information reaching the central nervous system rarely reaches consciousness under normal circumstances and when it does it produces only diffuse sensations like feelings of fullness or spasm.

The sensory endings in the viscera, unlike the majority of cutaneous receptors, have not been identified morphologically as showing receptor specializations. Instead, silver staining of the gut wall reveals numerous free nerve endings at three separate sites, and it is their location within the different layers of the gut wall which determines the receptor properties. Receptors in the mucosa, because of their proximity to the gut lumen, behave as chemoreceptors constantly monitoring the composition of gastrointestinal contents. They respond also to mechanical stimulation of the surface of the mucosa and so may detect the passage of solid food. The receptors within the muscle layers detect mechanical changes associated with contraction or stretch of the muscle itself while other receptors in the

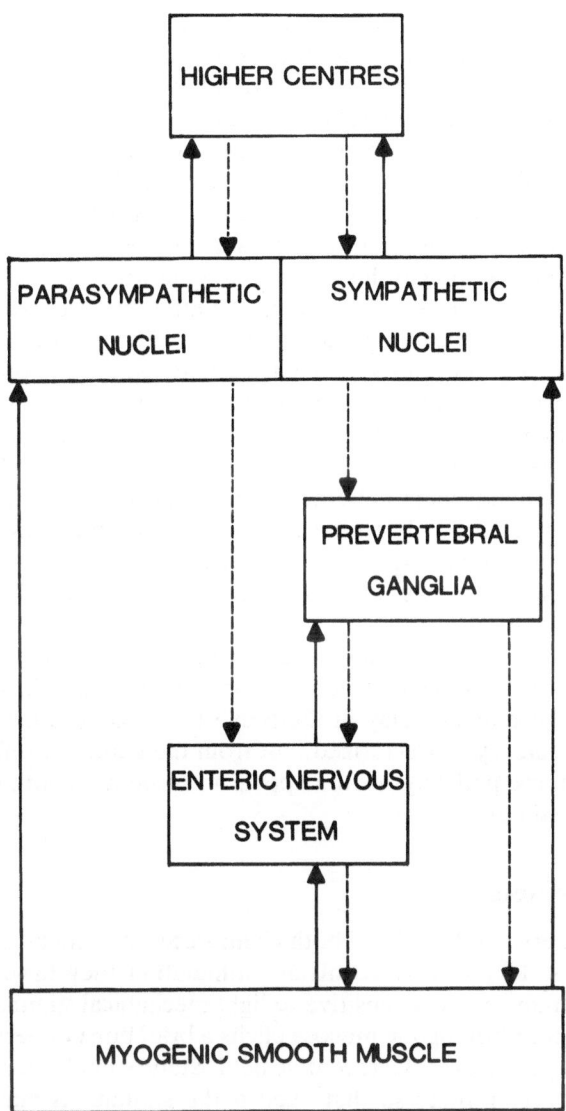

EXTRINSIC INNERVATION

HIGHER CENTRES

PARASYMPATHETIC NUCLEI

SYMPATHETIC NUCLEI

PREVERTEBRAL GANGLIA

ENTERIC NERVOUS SYSTEM

MYOGENIC SMOOTH MUSCLE

Figure 3.5 Schematic illustration of the hierarchy of nervous controls regulating gastrointestinal motility (Adapted from Davison, 1983)

serosal and mesenteric connections respond to movement or distortion of the viscera (Leek, 1977).

Evidence for these different receptor types stems from observations of reflex changes in digestive function associated with different stimuli. However, precise characterization of the receptors can only be achieved by direct electrophysiological recordings from individual afferent neurones.

One commonly used technique involves teasing slender filaments of nerve fibres from the whole nerve trunk and paring down until a small enough filament is obtained containing only one or a few viable afferent fibres. By placing the nerve strand on metal electrodes the nerve impulses travelling along these axons are detected as they pass over the recording site.

A second technique avoids the need for fine dissection of the nerve trunk by using microelectrodes which are inserted in the ganglion containing the cell bodies of the afferent fibres under investigation. Mei and his co-workers (see Mei, 1983) have applied this latter technique with great success to the vagal nodose ganglia. Here the cell bodies of afferent fibres from different organs appear to be grouped together; that is, there is viscerotopic organization, which enables areas of the ganglia containing afferent fibres from the abdominal viscera to be selected from other areas containing cardiovascular and respiratory neurones. Afferent fibres associated with mucosal and muscle receptors, but not serosal receptors, have been identified in the vagal and sacral parasympathetic nerves with the vagus being by far the most extensively studied. The serosal distortion receptors are associated with afferent fibres travelling in the splanchnic nerves and enter the spinal cord. Other basic differences are associated with the conduction velocities of action potentials in the two pathways. Vagal afferents are unmyelinated C fibres while the splanchnic nerves also contain small myelinated nerves and conduct impulses at higher velocities. Afferent neurones in the intramural plexuses whose axons relay in the prevertebral ganglia have not been electrophysiologically characterized, but from the nature of reflexes mediated through these pathways would appear to respond to both mechanical and chemical stimuli.

Mucosal receptors

The mucosal nerve endings have both chemoreceptive and mechanoreceptive properties. In the absence of any stimulation they have no resting discharge but they are very sensitive to light mechanical stimulation of the mucosal surface. Stroking the mucosa elicits a brief burst of nerve impulses as each stroke passes over the receptive field. Static stimuli elicit a response which adapts very rapidly so that even if the stimulus is maintained no further response is seen. These properties would suggest a role as contact receptors detecting the presence of solid or semisolid material within the lumen. However, in addition to this mechanical response, these receptors show maintained or slowly adapting responses to chemical stimulation (Figure 3.6). The majority of data, especially from earlier work, would suggest that these receptors are not specific to only one type of chemical stimulus. In most species the vagal mucosal receptors respond when both acidic and alkaline solutions flow over the receptive field. Only in the cat is there a separate population of receptors sensitive to either acidic or

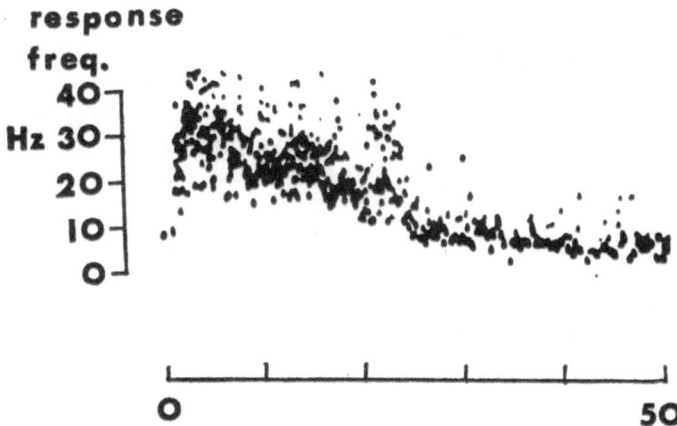

Figure 3.6 Response of a gastric chemoreceptor to irrigation of the receptive field with 0.1N hydrochloric acid. The record shows the instantaneous response frequency; each action potential generates a dot which is plotted according to the interval from the last action potential from which instantaneous frequency is calculated. Time is represented at the bottom in seconds (From Davison, 1972, with kind permission of the author and editor of Q. J. Exp. Physiol.)

alkaline pH. In the rat the receptors are even more non-specific and are also excited by such wide-ranging stimuli as water, alcohol and hypertonic sodium chloride. It is difficult, therefore, to ascribe specific functions to this type of afferent fibre although the sensitivity of duodenal sensory fibres to acid may implicate them in the feedback regulation of gastric emptying (see Chapter 6). More specific mucosal receptors have been described in the intestines; some respond only to monosaccharides especially glucose (Mei, 1978); others respond to mixtures of amino-acids (Jeanningros, 1982), while another class respond when hypotonic and hypertonic solutions are introduced into the lumen (Garnier and Mei, 1982). These more specific receptors may also play a role in the feedback regulation of gastric emptying, but may also be involved in the stimulation of postprandial motor activity in the small intestine (see Chapter 10) and in the regulation of food intake.

Muscle receptors

Vagal afferent recordings from mechanoreceptors in the oesophagus, stomach, small intestine and proximal colon have been described. These, unlike the mucosal receptors, are generally spontaneously active even when the viscus is empty and give a slowly adapting response to maintained distension of the viscus. In addition they are excited when a contraction, either spontaneous or evoked, passes over the receptive field. These mechanoreceptors, therefore, differ from the skeletal muscle spindle which, being parallel to the muscle fibres, only responds to stretch. Iggo (1955) coined the term 'in-series' tension receptor because they signal wall tension generated by both stretching and contraction. In the stomach a wide range of receptor sensitivity has been described. Some receptors have very low thresholds and respond to small changes in gastric volume causing minimal rises in intragastric pressure. Others have much higher thresholds and respond only when the stomach is grossly distended or undergoing powerful isometric contractions (Clarke and Davison, 1976).

Although, by definition, in-series tension receptors respond to both stretch and contraction, the primary stimulus to the receptor varies with their location within the gastrointestinal tract. The proximal stomach, for example, behaves as a distensible reservoir (see p. 94). Receptors in this region, therefore, respond as if they were volume receptors and show a

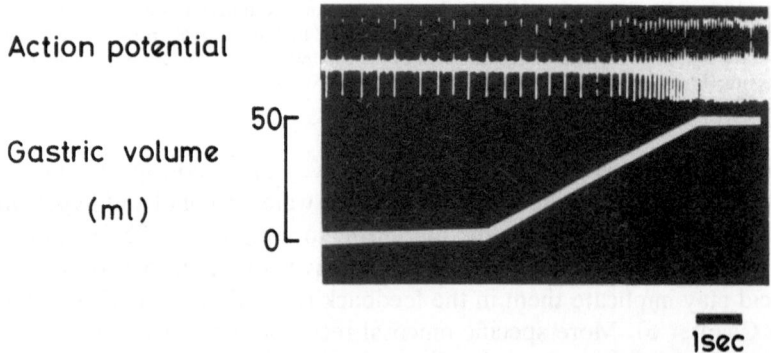

Action potential

Gastric volume

(ml)

50

0

1sec

Figure 3.7 Impulses in an afferent vagal fibre from a mechanoreceptor in the upper corpus. Upper trace, action potentials; lower trace, intragastric volume during a 50ml infusion of 0.9% NaCl (From Grundy and Scratcherd, 1984, with kind permission of the publisher, Praeger.)

discharge frequency proportional to the degree of distension (Figure 3.7). However. it must be remembered that these are indeed tension receptors and therefore an increase in volume associated with active relaxation of the stomach will cause a decrease in afferent firing. The antrum is a muscular pump which is not readily distensible. Receptors in this region are therefore stimulated primarily as each wave of contraction passes over the receptive field (Figure 3.8). Information from these receptors, and others in the oesophagus and intestine, is directed centrally regarding the amplitude and waveform of each visceral contraction.

Since many gastrointestinal reflexes are activated by distension and contraction of the viscera these receptors are likely to play an important role in the reflex regulation of motility. They may also be involved in the regulation of food intake since the lateral hypothalamus receives a mechanoreceptor input from both the stomach and intestine (Jeanningros, 1984).

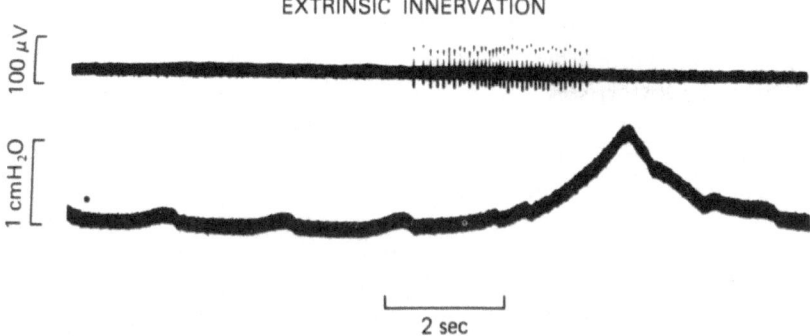

2 sec

Figure 3.8 Impulses in an afferent vagal fibre from a mechanoreceptor in the antrum. Upper trace, afferent nerve discharge; lower trace, intragastric pressure. As spontaneous waves of contraction pass over the receptive field, firing occurs in the afferent nerve. The three small transient waves on the intragastric pressure record were due to respiration (From Andrews, Grundy and Scratcherd, 1980b, with kind permission of the the editor of J. Physiol. (London))

Serosal receptors

These receptors have afferent fibres in the splanchnic nerves which enter the spinal cord at the same level as the sympathetic outflow and as such may be involved in sympathetic reflexes. Unlike the mucosal and muscle receptors which have a single receptive field, the serosal receptors have multiple receptive fields often over an area associated with more than one abdominal visceral organ (Figure 3.9). Single afferent fibres have been described which have as many as eight separate receptive fields distributed

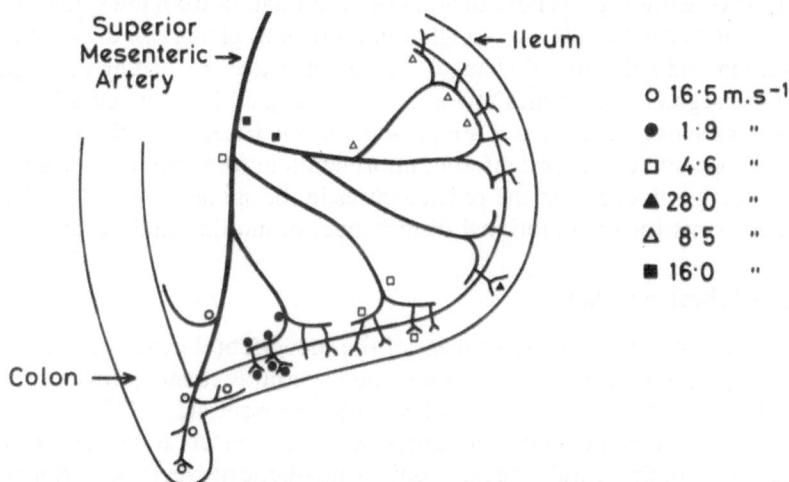

Figure 3.9 The receptive fields of six slowly adapting splanchnic mechanoreceptors associated with the ileum, ileocaecal junction and its mesentery. Each symbol represents one unit and the distribution of symbols shows the receptive fields. The values on the right refer to the afferent fibres conduction velocity (From Brooks, F. P. and Evers, P. W. *Nerves and the Gut*. (Thorofare, New Jersey: Slack Incorporated) © 1977, Slack Incorporated. Used by permission.)

along mesenteric arteries, at vascular divisions in the mesentery and on the walls of viscera (Morrison, 1977). As such they are less likely to be involved in the regulation of a single organ and more likely to have general effects on the whole tract. Recordings of afferent discharges reveal an irregular pattern of spike discharge due to the contributions from each of the separate receptor endings. At any one time the receptor generating the highest frequency of action potentials will dominate by antidromically invading the remaining terminals and colliding with their orthodromic impulses. The resulting discharge will therefore reflect this complexity. Distortion of the viscera is the effective stimulus to these receptors and as such they respond to movement of the viscera brought about by distension or contraction but not always reproducibly. Tension on the mesentery, and excessive distension, are painful stimuli, and the properties of splanchnic receptors suggests that they may be involved in mediating visceral pain. There is some evidence, however, for a more physiological role since the level of distension necessary to elicit a response in some splanchnic afferent fibres can be as low as that required to excite vagal afferent discharge.

REFLEX PATHWAYS

The afferent traffic entering the prevertebral ganglia, spinal cord and medulla can synaptically modify the efferent outflow back to the viscera thereby constituting a reflex. In addition, information from the spinal cord and medulla can be relayed to higher brain regions giving rise to conscious sensation and behavioural changes. Spinal anaesthesia reaching the upper thoracic segments abolishes abdominal visceral pain but not sensations of nausea or satiety; these latter are presumably mediated through the vagus. The integration of visceral afferent information in forebrain areas leads to descending influences on the reflex centres in the spinal cord and medulla and accounts for the emotional disturbances of motility that occur.

Prevertebral ganglia

Over the last few years the concept of the prevertebral ganglia have risen from mere relay stations on the sympathetic pathway to integrative centres for the control of the abdominal viscera (Szurszewski, 1977a; 1981b). Recordings from individual neurones in the prevertebral ganglia reveal inputs from both central (preganglionic sympathetic nerves) and peripheral sources. Considerable convergence from spinal inputs is evident from the multiple synaptic inputs from different spinal roots which summate with inputs from the viscera itself. There are also interconnections between adjacent prevertebral ganglia so that the capacity for integration is large. Recently, King and Szurszewski (1984) demonstrated that neurones in the inferior mesenteric ganglia receive an input from mechanoreceptors in the colon while neurones in the dorsal root ganglion do not. The authors concluded that mechanoreceptive information is referred mainly to the prevertebral ganglia with minimal involvement of the spinal cord.

Spinal cord

The observations described above together with earlier data demonstrating maintained sympathetic tone and maintained reflexes after decentralization of the prevertebral ganglia support the view that the sensory information in the splanchnic nerves entering the cord is primarily concerned with nociception. Further support for such a view can be inferred from the way this sensory information is relayed in the cord. Microelectrode recordings from second-order neurones in the thoracic spinal cord indicate that visceral afferent information and cutaneous afferent signals converge onto the same ascending spinal pathways (Cervero, 1983). In this study only 2% of the spinal neurones received an exclusively visceral afferent input. Visceral sensations are therefore predominantly mediated through convergent signals in the somatosensory pathways and presumably account for the phenomenon of referred pain. It is unlikely that these spinal neurones receiving convergent viscerocutaneous inputs are involved in specific reflexes regulating visceral function.

Sympathetic reflexes through the spinal cord have been described. Davison, Gradwell and Hersteinsson (1977) demonstrated electrophysiologically sympathetic spinal reflexes by electrically stimulating one branch of the colonic nerves while simultaneously recording from another branch. The evoked compound potential consisted of early and late phases with the latter progressively lost as the connections between the inferior mesenteric ganglia and spinal cord were sectioned. The compound response therefore consisted of a short latency response mediated through the ganglia and a longer latency response via the spinal cord. A physiological indication for such spinal reflexes is suggested from the observation that section of the splanchnic nerves or spinal anaesthesia generally results in the reduction of inhibitory sympathetic reflexes and an increase in gastrointestinal motor activity. However, because postganglionic sympathetic neurones receive an input from both the spinal cord and the periphery, removal of a tonic spinal input may well reduce transmission through the peripheral reflex arc.

Spinal reflexes associated with the sacral cord are more specific and their destruction depresses colonic motor activity. The defaecation reflex is stimulated by distension of the rectum and in spinal animals occurs without involvement of higher centres. Afferent discharge in the pelvic nerves reflexly excites the parasympathetic excitatory pathway to the colon and rectum and inhibits the tonic discharge in the motor nerves to the internal and external anal sphincters (see Chapter 8). The influence of higher centres on this reflex is evident in man who has voluntary control over the relaxation of the external anal sphincter.

Dorsomotor vagal nucleus

Considerable attention has been paid to reflexes whose afferent and efferent pathways lie in the vagus nerves. In 1959, Harper, Kidd and Scratcherd used electrical stimulation of the central end of one vagal branch to elicit a variety of reflex modifications of gastrointestinal motility and secretion. The efferent pathway was also in the vagus nerves and thereby constituted a vagovagal reflex. Neurophysiological analysis of this type of reflex involves recording the impulse traffic in the vagal pathway in response to stimuli which activate a specific type of visceral receptor, usually the in-series tension receptor. Observing the effect of a known sensory input on the activity of neurones in the vagal pathway through the brainstem provides a useful method of investigating the central organization of vagal reflexes. Recordings from the nucleus of the tractus solitarius or dorsomotor vagal nucleus require steriotaxically placed microelectrodes and subsequent histological verification of electrode positions to confirm the recording site. Additional techniques are also required to distinguish motoneurone from interneurone and rely on the phenomenon of 'collision' whereby antidromic action potentials, evoked by electrical stimulation of the vagus nerves, are cancelled out by spontaneous orthodromic action potentials when they collide and therefore fail to reach the recording electrode.

An alternative, less complicated, method is to record from the preganglionic fibres themselves as they travel in the vagus nerves to the abdomen and involves the dissection of slender nerve filaments from the intact vagal trunks. Both techniques are only applicable to anaesthetized animals. To get round this problem Miolan and Roman (see Roman and Gonella, 1981) have used an ingenious technique which allows indirect recording of vagal efferent activity from the conscious dog. The preparation depends on the reinnervation of the diaphragm by preganglionic vagal fibres following the anastomosis of the central end of one branch of the vagus in the thorax to the peripheral end of a severed phrenic nerve. The vagally reinnervated hemidiaphragm is then transplanted to a subcutaneous site so that electrical recordings can be made from needle electrodes inserted into diaphragmatic muscle. A spike is recorded each time an action potential in the vagal fibre innervating that particular muscle cell reaches the diaphragm and so provides a means of recording vagal activity indirectly in the conscious animal. A similar technique has been used to study the vagal efferent fibres supplying the proximal oesophagus, but in these studies the left vagus nerve was sutured to the left spinal accessory nerve and electrical activity recorded from the sternocleidomastoideus and trapezius muscles (Roman and Tieffenbach, 1972).

One thing lacking from all these studies is information on the precise target destination of individual nerve fibres. This can only be inferred from the temporal relationship between the neurone's discharge pattern and the gastrointestinal event under investigation and from the nature of afferent inputs it receives. As a consequence of these limitations, electrophysiological studies have concentrated on reflexes which regulate gastric and oesophageal motility. This is because these regions receive a higher proportion of the vagal innervation, and so statistically efferent fibres destined for these regions are more likely to be found. No definitive study of intestinal reflexes have been made although efferent fibres destined for these more distal regions are probably included in other studies of gastric regulation.

The general feature of the vagal efferent activity in monogastric animals, as opposed to ruminants which have a compound stomach, is that the majority of efferent neurones are spontaneously active. There is an irregular, low frequency discharge which is generated centrally since it continues, albeit at a different frequency, when the vagal afferent input is removed. The change in discharge frequency after vagotomy is a consequence of removing the tonic afferent input which can either enhance or inhibit the centrally generated efferent discharge. These excitatory and inhibitory processes within the brainstem become more evident as the frequency of action potentials in afferent fibres is increased. Thus gastric distension which activates the in-series tension receptors will reflexly excite some vagal efferent neurones while simultaneously suppressing, or completely inhibiting, the discharge of others (Figure 3.10). Waves of contraction also activate the tension receptors giving rise to phasic changes in afferent impulse traffic which, because of reflex connections in the brainstem, result in a phasic pattern of efferent activity. However, since contractions activate higher threshold afferent fibres the potential for more complex patterns of efferent discharge arise (Figure 3.11). In the simplest case low and high threshold afferent fibres have the same central effect, either excitation or inhibition, so that the efferent fibre reflects this and is similarly either excited or inhibited by both distension and contraction. In the more complex situation, low and high threshold afferent fibres have the opposite effect of efferent firing so that a particular response to distension may be reversed as the level of distension increases further or when contractions occur (see Figure 3.11).

The most striking feature of this grouping of efferent discharge patterns is that they form two distinct pairs with the activity in one of the pairs being modified in the opposite direction to the other. This suggests that the neurones in the vagal nucleus are reciprocally organized so that as the discharge of one group of neurones is enhanced another group is simultaneously suppressed. Since the vagus nerve contains two motor pathways to

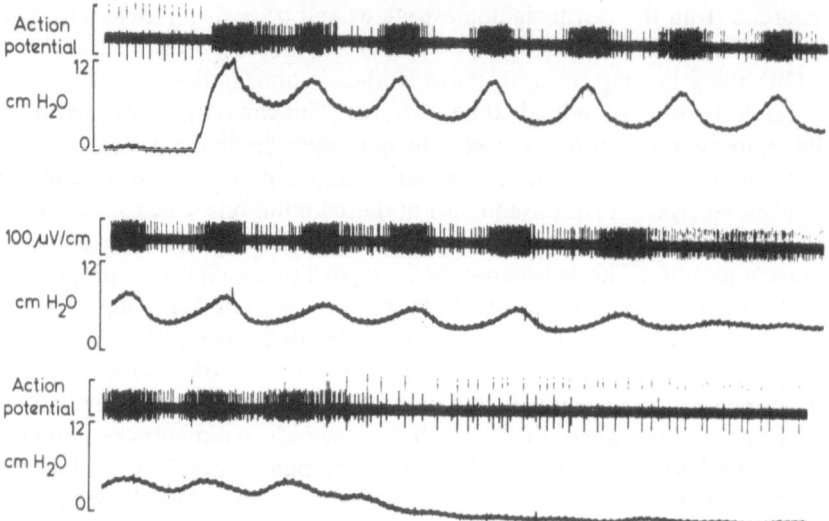

Figure 3.10 Impulses in two vagal efferent neurones recorded simultaneously from the same nerve strand in response to gastric distension. A 4 min continuous recording is shown: upper trace, efferent nerve discharge; lower trace, intragastric pressure. One efferent neurone was spontaneous active and was inhibited during gastric distension with 40ml 0.9% NaCl. A second efferent neurone with action potentials of slightly lower amplitude than the first was recruited upon distension and discharged phasically in rhythm with the fluctuations in intragastric pressure due to antral contractions (From Scratcherd and Grundy, 1982, with kind permission of the publisher, Raven Press)

the gastrointestinal tract, one excitatory and the other inhibitory, the observation of reciprocally modulated pairs of vagal neurones might indicate that activation of vagovagal reflexes, either excitatory or inhibitory, is accompanied by concomitant inhibition of the antagonistic pathway (Figure 3.12).

Convergence of afferent information onto the dorsomotor vagal nucleus is considerable. Efferent activity can be influenced by a wide range of different stimuli applied to the oesophagus, stomach and intestine. Investigations into the extent of this afferent convergence help to clarify the potential destination of individual efferent fibres in terms of the reflexes in which they are involved. For example, the discharge of efferent neurones innervating the lower oesophageal sphincter will be temporally related to the opening and closing of the sphincter irrespective of the stimuli involved. Using this approach Miolan and Roman (1978a and b) have described the characteristics of efferent neurones destined for different regions of the gastrointestinal tract, especially those to the lower oesophageal sphincter and stomach where again reciprocal modulation of excitatory and inhibitory pathways is proposed (see Chapters 5 and 6).

The convergence of afferent inputs onto individual efferent fibres must be considerable if only in terms of numbers. There is also functional

EXTRINSIC INNERVATION

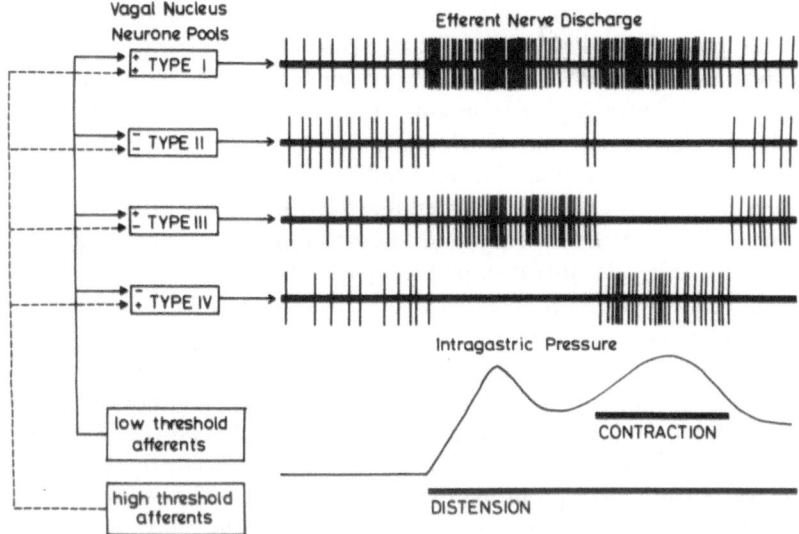

Figure 3.11 Reflex modulation of vagal preganglionic fibres by inputs from vagal afferent fibres. Low threshold afferent fibres are activated by both distension and contraction. High threshold afferent fibres are activated mainly during contraction (From data by Davison and Grundy, 1978, and modified from Davison, 1983)

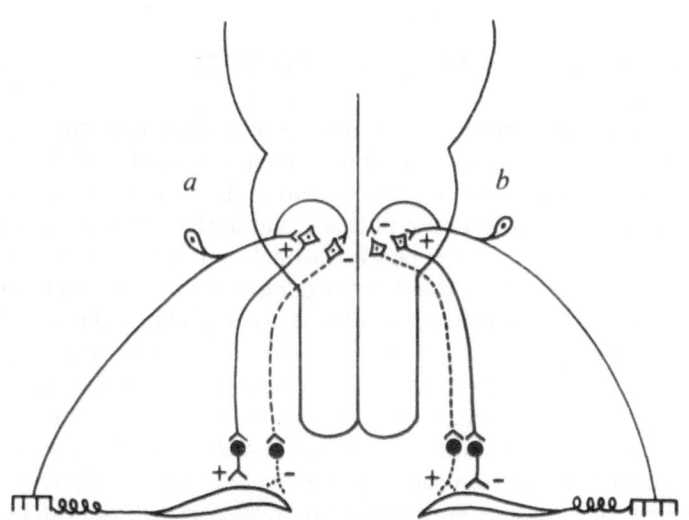

Figure 3.12 Schematic representation of the central organization of vago-vagal reflexes. A is an excitatory and B an inhibitory reflex. In each case, vagal afferent fibres activate the appropriate excitatory (+) or inhibitory (−) pathway. In addition there is reciprocal inhibition of the antagonist pathway (dotted line). For simplicity the reflexes are shown as monosynaptic and the afferent fibres as dividing onto both pathways (From Davison, 1983, with kind permission of the author and publisher, Wright, PSG)

53

evidence for convergence. Efferent fibres can be influenced by various stimuli applied to a wide area of the gastrointestinal tract. The same preganglionic vagal fibre can therefore provide the efferent limb of a range of vagovagal reflexes and may account for the relatively low number of such fibres. Convergence from afferent pathways travelling up the spinal cord has also been described (Grundy, Salih and Scratcherd, 1981). Duodenal and colonic distension has a predominantly inhibitory effect on vagal efferent activity and at the same time suppresses gastrointestinal motility. While the peripheral effect is in part mediated through sympathetic noradrenergic pathways, there may also be simultaneous inhibition of the preganglionic vagal innervation.

The information relayed through the nucleus of the tractus solitarius converges on the dorsomotor vagal nucleus where there is either excitation or inhibition of the preganglionic neurone. Central processing is therefore fairly simple and merely serves to set levels reciprocally in the vagal excitatory and inhibitory pathways to the viscera. In animals with compound stomach the central organization is much more complex. Here both 'rate' and 'form and amplitude' circuits have been postulated to control the periodicity and discharge frequency of the vagal efferent supply (Harding and Leek, 1972). The efferent fibres innervating different regions of the reticulorumen are then activated in turn to coordinate their complex contractions.

INFLUENCES FROM HIGHER BRAIN REGIONS

If the importance of extrinsic nerves in controlling gastrointestinal motility has been questioned then there must be even more doubt as to the role of higher brain centres in physiological regulation. However, given that local integration within the intramural plexuses and in the reflex centres in the spinal cord and brainstem can cope with normal circumstances, the function of the forebrain is to adjust these lower controls so that visceral function can be maintained in a state of readiness to respond to the necessities imposed by changes in both internal and external environment. Because of the delicate perceptions of the central nervous system and the varied emotional states that ensue, such things as an unpleasant sight, anxiety over an impending examination, or charged emotions like anger and fear can have immediate and profound effects on the viscera. Hypermotility and atony are the two extremes of motility responses to emotional states.

The additional integrative features of the central nervous system are required for the processes of swallowing, vomiting and defaecation which all depend on coordination between autonomically controlled smooth muscle and skeletal muscle controlled by somatic nerves. Bilateral 'swallowing centres' in the medulla oblongata control the sequential activation of the different muscle groups in the mouth, pharynx and oesophagus whose contractions direct food towards the stomach (see Chapter 5). Swallowing is normally reflexly induced following stimulation of taste buds and receptors lining the buccal cavity. Since swallowing can also be initiated voluntarily, the medullary centres must also receive descending influences from as far up as the cerebral cortex.

Similarly, defaecation depends on a sacral spinal reflex which in man is subjected to higher control. Spinal section results in impaired defaecation initially because of spinal shock which causes flaccid anal sphincters and an impaired reflex response to rectal distension together with paralysis of the abdominal muscles that participate in the voluntary expulsion of faeces. Later the sacral cord regains autonomic control due to the recovery of the spinal reflexes. However, there is no subjective urge to defaecate and no cortical participation in when and where defaecation takes place.

Vomiting also depends on coordination between autonomic and somatic control of smooth and skeletal muscle. Here there is relaxation of the stomach and lower oesophageal sphincter and simultaneous contraction of the abdominal muscles and diaphragm so that gastric contents are forced out of the flaccid stomach. The trigger to vomit can arise from a number of independent sources. Afferent impulses from the gastrointestinal tract travelling in both the vagal and splanchnic nerves can elicit vomiting. There is also a chemical trigger zone in the brainstem responding to emetics in the blood. Vomiting can also result from unpleasant psychological factors or from stimulation of the vestibular apparatus, as during motion sickness.

Another illustration of the relationship between the abdominal viscera and the forebrain stems from the association between appetite, hunger, satiety and the intake of food on the one hand and the gastrointestinal tract on the other. The lateral and ventromedial nuclei of the hypothalamus are important in these functions and receive inputs from vagal afferent fibres. These areas are also implicated in the motor response to cephalic stimuli in much the same way as gastric secretion is stimulated by the sight, smell and taste of food (see p. 164).

From this brief outline, it would seem that many brain areas receive inputs from visceral afferents. Indeed, the abdominal viscera are represented in the somatosensory cortex. Many forebrain areas also have descending projections which ultimately synapse on the preganglionic neural cell bodies of the parasympathetic and sympathetic nuclei. It will come as no surprise, therefore, to discover that electrical stimulation of almost any brain region has an effect on gastrointestinal motility (Eliasson, 1960). These widespread connections make mapping of autonomic connections in the brain and spinal cord difficult. It is even more difficult, however, to reach conclusions on the generation and spread of autonomic impulses that occur under normal conditions.

Other forms of neural mapping involve the use of tracer substances that are taken up by nerve terminals and transported back to the neural cell body. Localization of one such substance, horseradish peroxidase, has confirmed the importance of the reticular formation and hypothalamus as integrative stations for visceral control. The reticular formation is a network of interneurones occupying the midline of the brain between the medulla and thalamus. It is important in distributing visceral information centrally but also receives converging descending impulses which can influence the somatosensory ascending pathways in the cord.

The hypothalamus is the principal site for integration within the central visceral pathways. Two nuclei are of prime importance as illustrated by the pronounced visceral responses to electrical stimulation of these regions. Stimulation of anterior hypothalamic nuclei enhance gastrointestinal motility via parasympathetic pathways, while stimulation of the nuclei that lie posteriorly and laterally are associated with the sympathetic outflow. Cerebral mechanisms interact with the hypothalamus via parts of the limbic system, especially the hippocampus and amygdala. The limbic system exerts modulatory influences on behaviour and is responsible for the emotional disturbances of gastrointestinal function.

There is therefore a hierarchy of both peripheral and central controls influencing gastrointestinal motility. As one passes from the intramural plexuses, through the reflex centres in the prevertebral ganglia, spinal cord and medulla, and on through the brain, there is an expanding network of interneurones which provides the means for ever-increasing possibilities of interaction.

4
Neurocrines, endocrines and paracrines

INTRODUCTION

The regulation of gastrointestinal muscle contractility is brought about by a complex interplay between a wide range of endogenous chemical modulators. Classically, two routes for regulation exist. Neurotransmitters are released from nerve axons that lie in close proximity to their target cells. Hormones are blood-borne messengers distributed to all peripheral tissue, but they have specific actions only on cells with the appropriate receptors. An additional route lies midway between neurotransmitter and hormone and is provided by substances which are released into the interstitial space and act as 'local hormones' or 'paracrines' (Figure 4.1).

Recent technical developments allowing chemical modulators to be detected and visualized have led to a great upsurge in interest in peptide messengers. Radioimmunoassay and immunohistochemistry utilize radiolabelled or dye-labelled antibodies raised against a particular sequence of aminoacids or tertiary protein structure. When the antibody binds its 'specific' antigen, the peptide is marked and its concentration can be estimated, or its localization in specific cells identified. These techniques, however, are fraught with difficulties and require careful interpretation. Not least of the problems is the need to characterize the specificity of the antibody so that cross-reactions with peptides which have similarities in their aminoacid sequences are minimized. For this reason, the detection of these antibodies is referred to, for example with gastrin, as gastrin-like immunity to acknowledge possible contributions from similar peptides. To establish with certainty the presence of a substance in a particular tissue, the peptide must be extracted and either its aminoacid sequence determined or its structure established using sensitive chromatographic techniques. Developments in these techniques have paralleled the interest in regulatory peptides.

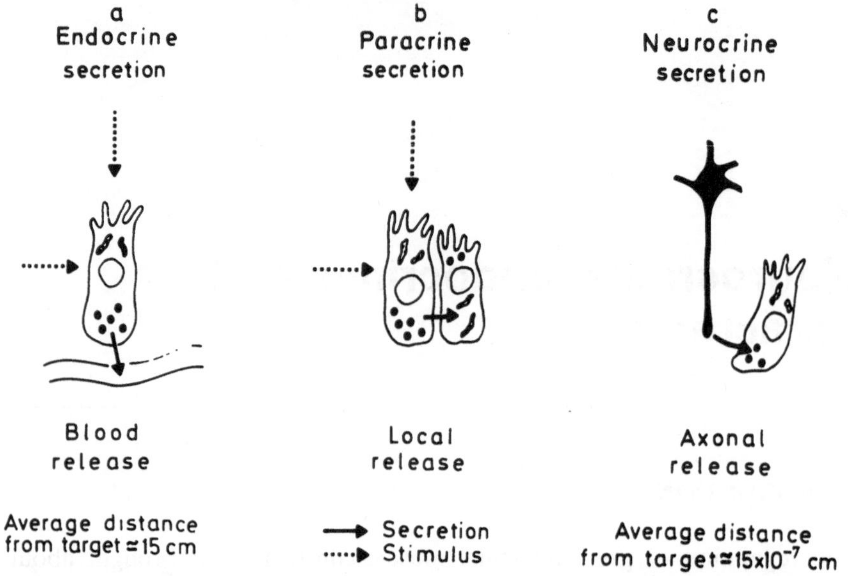

a
Endocrine
secretion

b
Paracrine
secretion

c
Neurocrine
secretion

Blood
release

Local
release

Axonal
release

Average distance
from target ≅ 15 cm

——▶ Secretion
·····▶ Stimulus

Average distance
from target ≅ 15x10^{-7} cm

Figure 4.1 Diagrammatic representation of the mode of delivery of substances acting as gut hormones **a**, paracrine messengers **b**, or neurotransmitters **c** (From Bertaccini, 1982, with kind permission of the author and publisher, Springer–Verlag)

Three important implications for physiology, and gastrointestinal physiology in particular, have arisen from this type of study. First, an enormous variety of peptides have been identified within the various layers of the gut wall. In the mucosa these exist within a widespead endocrine system while a great variety of peptides are also found within neural elements of the intramural nerves. Second, peptides originally considered to be hormones have been identified within nervous elements of the intramural plexuses where they may act as neurotransmitters. Third, nerves have been shown to contain and release more than one transmitter.

The duplicity of function of certain 'regulatory peptides', acting as both hormone and transmitter, is not restricted to the enteric nervous system. Many of the 'gut hormones' have been identified in the brain and spinal cord where again they may play a role in nervous transmission (Dockray and Gregory, 1980). For example, the C-terminal octapeptide of CCK is found throughout the central and enteric nervous system while the full CCK-33 molecule is released from the gut mucosa into the bloodstream during the course of a meal and controls pancreatic and biliary flow into the intestines. In other examples the same molecular form has both endocrine and neurocrine functions. The distinction between hormone and transmitter substances is therefore becoming blurred especially when some have been identified additionally as paracrines.

The widespread distribution of these peptides in both the CNS and gastrointestinal tract has led to the collective term 'brain–gut peptides' to illustrate their principal locality in these two sites. A more far-reaching term, 'brain–gut axis', has entered the literature which implies a special interrelationship between the functioning of peptides from these two sites with regard to gastrointestinal control. However, one of the richest sources of CCK-8 is the cerebral cortex, an area which has little to do with gastrointestinal control.

The detection within neurones or mucosal endocrine cells cannot, on its own, conclusively establish specific roles as transmitter or hormone. Other criteria – to establish storage in cytoplasmic organelles, release by specific stimuli and actions on specific membrane receptors – must be satisfied. In this chapter, the nature and variety of endogenous messengers and the evidence for their involvement in the regulation of gastrointestinal motility are discussed.

NEUROMUSCULAR TRANSMISSION

The neural control of gastrointestinal musculature is mainly one of modulation of a myogenic syncytium of smooth muscle cells rather than the absolute neurogenic control of skeletal muscle. As a consequence the innervation of the two types of muscle is markedly different (see Burnstock, 1979; 1981).

(1) The innervation of smooth muscle is relatively sparse, especially in the longitudinal muscle layer, with very few cells receiving direct connections from nerve fibres.

(2) There is no specialized endplate on smooth muscle cells and the junctional cleft varies in length from tissue to tissue. In circular muscle small gaps of approximately 20 nm between nerve and muscle are common, while in longitudinal muscle long diffusion paths of over 100 nm are the norm. The released transmitter will therefore spread over a wide area and affect many cells.

(3) The transmitter is not released from nerve fibre endings but from varicose regions of the nerve axon that occur at 5–10 μm intervals (Figure 4.2A). Vesicles within the varicosities contain the transmitter substance which is released *en passage* as the action potential conducts along the nerve axon (Figure 4.2B). Transmitter release is not, therefore, restricted to a small area of muscle.

The essential feature of this innervation is simultaneous modulation of many smooth muscle cells which behave as a single unit because of electrotonic coupling through the low-resistance gap-junction. Although the long diffusion path for transmitter action will mean that junctional transmission is slow compared to that in skeletal muscle, this is not a particular disadvantage to the slowly contracting visceral muscle.

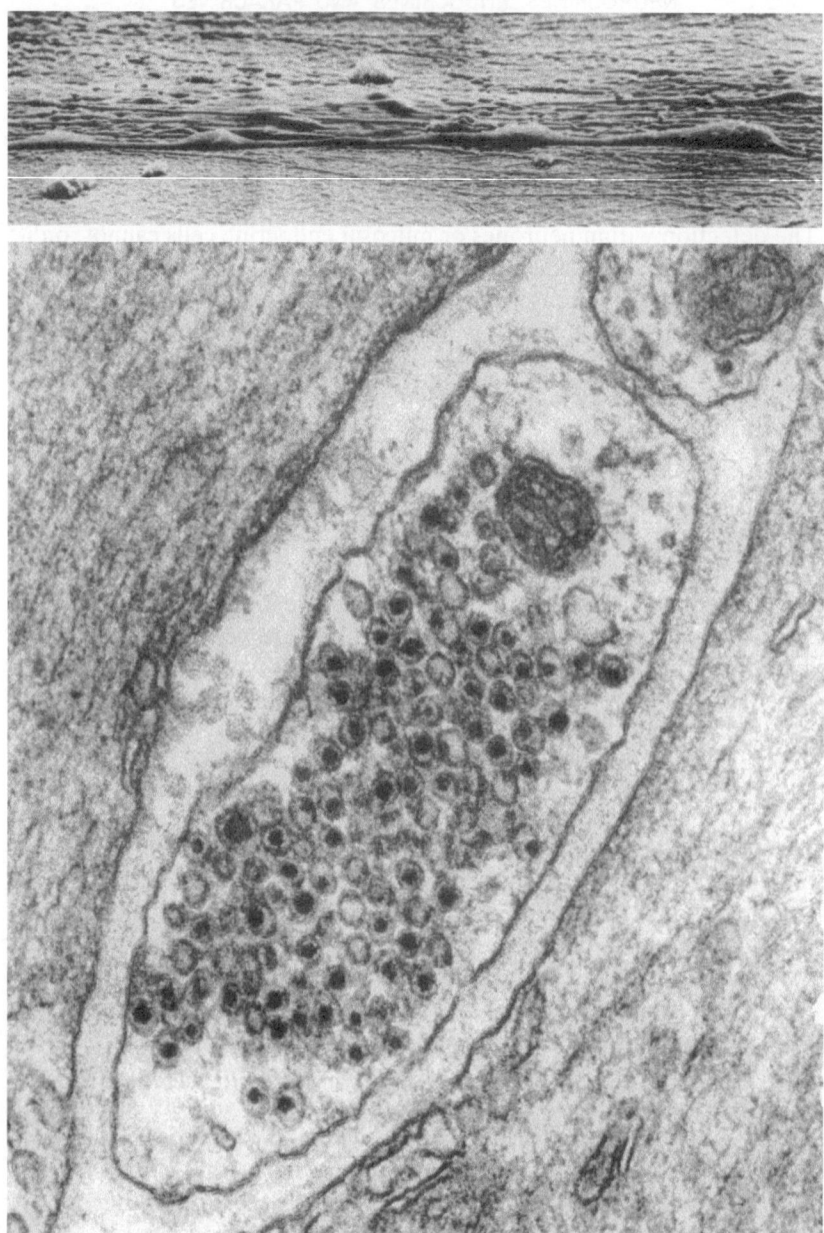

Figure 4.2 A: Scanning electron micrograph of varicosities in a single nerve fibre growing in a culture of newborn guinea-pig sympathetic ganglia. Photographed at an angle of 70° and magnified 5340×. (From Burnstock, 1975, with kind permission of the author and publisher, Plenum Publishing Corporation.) **B:** Transmission electron micrograph of a section through a sympathetic nerve varicosity. Note the vesicles of stored neurotransmitter, the wide and variable cleft and the absence of postjunctional specialization (magnified 48000×) (From Furness *et al.*, with the kind permission of the authors and the editor of J. Pharmacol. Exp. Ther. © (1970))

Excitatory transmission

The main excitatory neuromuscular transmitter in the gastrointestinal tract is acetylcholine (ACh). This is released from enteric nerves innervating both longitudinal and circular muscle layers, and the contractile effect of this release can be blocked by muscarinic antagonists like the belladonna alkaloid, atropine. Parasympathetic nerve stimulation also releases ACh from one population of postganglionic fibres which appear to provide the final common pathway for reflexes mediated locally through the enteric nervous system and extrinsic parasympathetic reflexes (Langley, 1921).

The synaptic events at cholinergic nerves have been well characterized. ACh is synthesized in the neural cell body and terminal axon by choline acetyltransferase. It is stored in electron-transparent agranular vesicles within the nerve varicosities and released by exocytosis during conduction of a nerve impulse. The postjunctional permeability changes resulting in membrane depolarization are brought about by the interaction of ACh with muscarinic receptors. Inactivation is mainly achieved locally by the enzyme, acetylcholinesterase, found near the postjunctional membrane.

After blockade of cholinergic transmission with atropine, a contractile response can be elicited in *in vitro* segments of small and large intestine by transmural electrical stimulation, and *in vivo* by vagal and pelvic nerve stimulation (Collman, Grundy and Scratcherd, 1984a; Fasth, Hulten and Nordgren, 1980). The nature of this non-cholinergic transmitter is not yet resolved but is not noradrenaline. The two best candidates at present are the indoleamine 5-hydroxytryptamine (5-HT) and the peptide substance P.

Neurones containing substanceP have been identified immunohistochemically in the myenteric plexus, and nerve fibres run orally and aborally into the adjacent circular muscle layer. It is released by nerve stimulation and is a potent stimulator of muscle contraction by both a direct action on the muscle and by indirect actions within the ganglia. The widespread distribution of substance P-containing neurones would suggest they play more than one regulatory role with separate classes of neurones fulfilling different functions.

There is also abundant evidence implicating 5-HT as the excitatory transmitter, but because of its diverse actions on interneurones there is considerable uncertainty with respect to neuromuscular transmission (see below, p. 70).

Inhibitory transmitter

As mentioned in the last chapter, noradrenaline is not the main inhibitory transmitter to the gastrointestinal muscle layers. Noradrenergic fibres can be visualized following staining using the Falck–Hillarp technique and the varicose nerve fibres are seen mainly around the intramural ganglia although a few run into the muscle layers (Figure 4.3). These noradrenergic

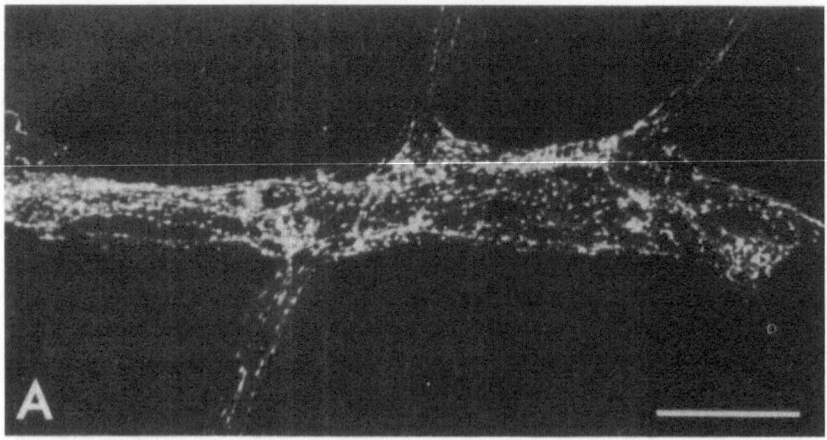

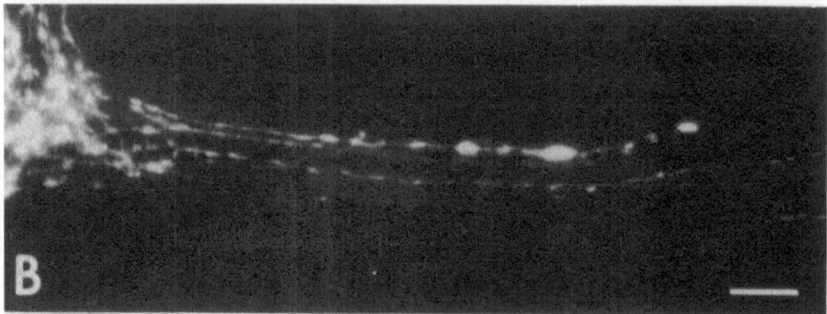

Figure 4.3 Fluorescence microscopy for catecholamines. Myenteric plexus of the guinea-pig ileum. **A**: A large ganglion and its connecting strands. The fluorescent axons are varicose and form an intricate mesh around ganglion neurones (these appear as dark areas since they do not contain catecholamines). Marker: $100\,\mu$m. **B**: Fluorescent fibres running in a connecting strand. Marker: $20\,\mu$m. (From Gabella, 1979b, with kind permission of the author and the publisher, Academic Press.)

nerve fibres are not of intrinsic origin since they disappear following extrinsic denervation. The hyperpolarization of smooth muscle cells during electrical stimulation of the paravascular nerve bundles involves both alpha and beta adrenoreceptors and occurs only after prolonged periods of high frequency stimulation (Figure 4.4a). This response is suggested to result from overspill of noradrenaline from the nearby ganglia. Stimulation of the intrinsic inhibitory nerves, on the otherhand, produces sharp inhibitory junction potentials even with single stimuli (see Figure 4.4b). In sphincteric regions noradrenaline causes contraction via a mechanism involving the alpha-adrenoreceptor while beta-receptor activation is again inhibitory. As will be discussed below (p. 69) noradrenaline from sympathetic origin primarily acts on the ganglia where it inhibits transmission in the parasympathetic cholinergic pathway.

The inhibitory nervous pathways of intrinsic origin are found along the

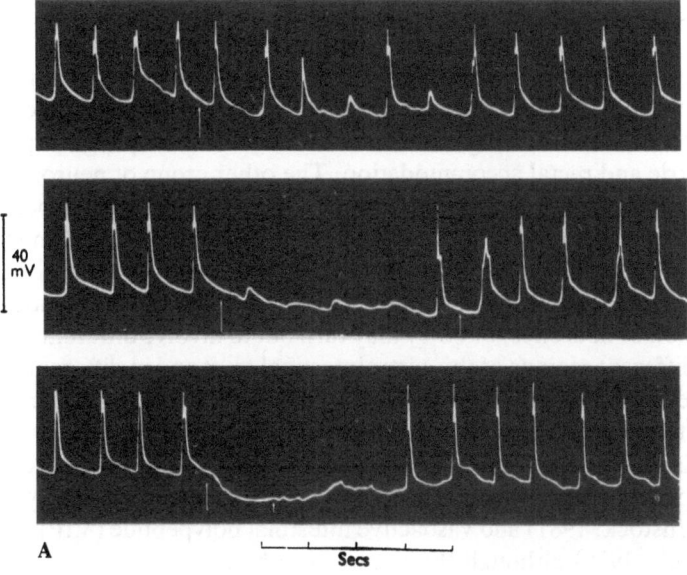

40
mV

A

Secs

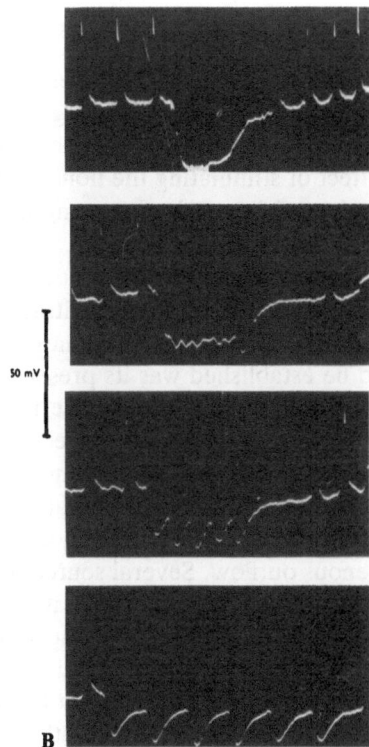

50 mV

B

Secs

Figure 4.4 Comparison of the effect of sympathetic nerve stimulation and transmural electrical stimulation on the membrane potential of guinea-pig taenia coli. A: sympathetic stimulation (during arrows) at 4, 10 and 60 pulses s^{-1} causes a progressively larger hyperpolarization and inhibition of spontaneous spikes. B: transmural stimulation at (from the bottom upwards) 1, 2, 4, and 60 pulses s^{-1} evokes pronounced hyperpolarizations even with single pulses (From Bennett *et al.*, 1966a and b, with kind permission of the authors and the editor of J. Physiol. (London))

entire length of the gastrointestinal tract where they mainly innervate the circular muscle layer and are involved in two main events. One group of intrinsic inhibitory nerves receives a preganglionic input from the parasympathetic vagal and pelvic supply and is important in receptive relaxation associated with swallowing, relaxation of the lower oesophageal sphincter, and gastric and rectal accommodation. The other group of neurones mediates the descending wave of inhibition which precedes intestinal peristalsis. Both cause muscle relaxation by hyperpolarizing the muscle cell membrane but they have different characteristics relating to the time course of events. There is a tendency to view the inhibitory nerves as an homogeneous population of neurones, but they may turn out to involve different transmitters in different regions of the gastrointestinal tract and in different species.

There has been considerable speculation as to the nature of the inhibitory transmitter. Dopamine and bradykinin have been suggested but the evidence is flimsy. The most likely candidates at present are adenosine triphosphate (ATP) and related purines, Burnstock's purinergic hypothesis (see Burnstock, 1981) and vasoactive intestinal polypeptide (VIP) (Fahrenkrug *et al.*, 1978) although there may be others.

The purinergic hypothesis

The basis for this hypothesis followed the discovery of an inhibitory innervation of the guinea-pig taenia coli (see p. 129) that was not blocked by cholinergic or adrenergic antagonists. ATP was found to mimic the effect of stimulating the non-adrenergic, non-cholinergic inhibitory nerves and was followed by a systematic series of experiments to satisfy the criteria for a neurotransmitter.

The main problems that needed to be overcome related to the ubiquitous distribution of ATP as an intracellular source of energy. Thus all cells will contain ATP and the enzymes responsible for its synthesis. What needed to be established was its presence in nerve terminals packaged in vesicles ready for subsequent release into the extracellular space around smooth muscle cells. Tritium-labelled adenosine has been shown to be actively taken up by segments of stomach and intestine and stored as tritiated ATP in nerves. Following electrical stimulation of the nerves the ATP is released and its breakdown products, adenosine and inosine, can be detected in the venous outflow. Several sources of this ATP, other than that postulated to be release from inhibitory nerves terminals exists. ATP released from nerve fibres during the conduction of action potentials, or from muscle as it responds to nerve stimulation have been largely eliminated as a potential source. What is more dificult to exclude is ATP that may be released from nerve terminals along with other, more established, neurotransmitters like acetylcholine or noradrenaline. However, much more ATP is released by stimulation of non-adrenergic, non-cholinergic nerves than when, for example, the sympathetic nerves are stimulated.

The major approach to the investigation of purinergic transmission is pharmacological, whereby mimickry between the action of ATP and inhibitory nerve stimulation are compared. Drug treatments which modify both these simultaneously support the hypothesis, while modification of one without the other would not be consistent with ATP as the transmitter.

Tissue from the gastrointestinal tract of rodents and lagomorphs show a close correlation between nerve-mediated relaxations and those associated with the exogenous application of ATP. In gastrointestinal segments from cat, dog, pig and ferret, ATP can have the opposite effect to nerve-mediated relaxations. However, where mimickry does occur it can be very close (Figure 4.5), not only in direction and time course of response but also in the membrane events (hyperpolarization) associated with it. A consistent finding with both inhibitory nerve stimulation and ATP application is that a secondary aftercontraction often follows the relaxation especially when the prevailing tone is low (see Figure 4.5). This contraction generally occurs as the stimulus is switched off and is called a 'rebound contraction'. The presence of a rebound contraction has consequently tended to be used as additional evidence for purinergic transmission, although some tissues in which ATP is unlikely to be the transmitter still show rebounds. Burnstock considers that rebound contractions arise because ATP stimulates prostaglandin production which then contracts the muscle. As such, rebounds can be prevented by pretreating preparations with indomethacin, an agent which prevents the enzymatic synthesis of prostaglandins.

Repeated applications of large doses of ATP or its long lasting analogues cause a diminution of effect (tachyphylaxis) so that eventually a condition is reached where no response can be mediated. A parallel reduction in nerve-mediated responses in appropriate preparations again indicate ATP as the transmitter.

Specific antagonists of ATP action have not been identified but two groups of compounds are reported to have the same effect on nerve-mediated and exogenous ATP responses leading to the suggestion that two types of purinergic receptor exist. P^1 receptors are most sensitive to adenosine and antagonized by methylxanthines, while P^2 receptors respond more readily to ATP and are antagonized by quinidine, 2-substituted imidazolines, 2,2'-pyridylisatogen and apamin (an extract from bee venom). P^2 receptors are predominant on gastrointestinal smooth muscle while P^1 receptors appear to be presynaptic receptors modifying transmitter release.

The purinergic hypothesis, like all good hypotheses, has stimulated a great deal of interest and an enormous amount of data both for and against ATP as the inhibitory transmitter. Taken as a whole, there is reasonable evidence in favour of ATP as the non-adrenergic, non-cholinergic transmit-

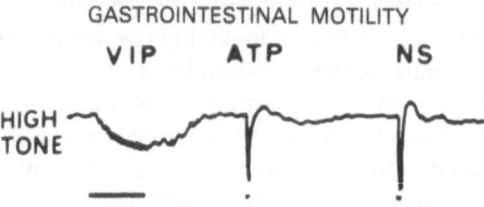

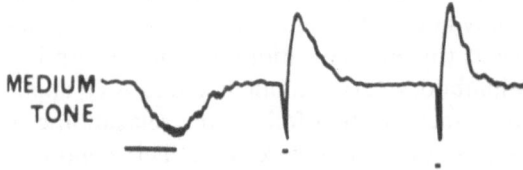

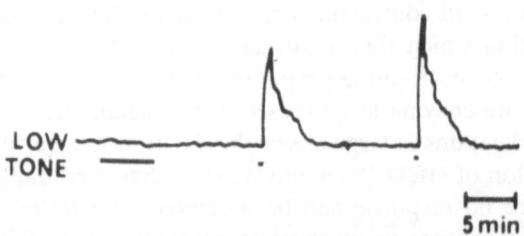

Figure 4.5 Comparison of the inhibitory responses of the guinea-pig taenia coli to VIP $(0.5\mu g\,ml^{-1})$, ATP $(0.5\mu g\,ml^{-1})$ and nerve stimulation (NS: 0.2 ms duration pulses delivered at 5Hz and supramaximal voltage for 30 s) in high, medium and low tone preparations. Atropine $(1\mu g\,ml^{-1})$ and guanethidine $(1\mu g\,ml^{-1})$ were present throughout (From Cocks and Burnstock, 1979, with kind permission of the authors and the editor of Eur. J. Pharmacol.)

ter to gastrointestinal smooth muscle in rat, guinea-pig and rabbit. A few question marks still exist not least because there is also good evidence for VIP as the inhibitory transmitter especially in the carnivore gut.

The peptidergic (VIP) hypothesis

The location of VIP within intramural nerve elements has been demonstrated immunohistochemically. The immunoreactive cell bodies are located in both the myenteric and submucosal plexuses and in numerous axons supplying the circular muscle layer especially of the sphincteric regions. Following damage to myenteric continuity, VIP accumulates on the oral side of a lesion and disappears on the anal side suggesting that the VIP neurones project aborally to the circular muscle layer, an observation consistent with involvement in descending inhibition.

VIP-like immunoreactivity in the venous effluent from the stomach increases during electrical stimulation of the vagal non-adrenergic, non-cholinergic pathway, and also during reflex activation of the inhibitory pathway by oesophageal distension. On the other hand, injection of VIP causes relaxation of gastrointestinal smooth muscle. The slowness of the guinea-pig taenia coli response to VIP in Figure 4.5 is taken as evidence against VIP as the non-adrenergic, non-cholinergic transmitter to this tissue. Other evidence concerning the selective inhibition of this tissue's response to nerve stimulation and ATP while leaving the VIP response unaffected would support this conclusion. However, in other tissues the nerve-mediated inhibition is equally slow and long-lasting. Gastric relaxation in response to vagal stimulation is one such example. In the cat and ferret the gastric relaxation following VIP infusion is remarkable in its similarity to the nerve-mediated response (Figure 4.6) – a point which highlights the possibility of more than one inhibitory transmitter.

Like ATP, no specific antagonists to VIP exist. However, nerve-mediated and VIP-mediated relaxations of the lower oesophageal sphincter were reduced by treating with antibodies raised to VIP while relaxations mediated by noradrenaline remained unaffected (Goyal, Said and Rattan, 1979).

Evidence is therefore accumulating in favour of VIP as the inhibitory transmitter to certain tissues of some species, while ATP is more likely to be the transmitter in other tissues from other species. Great rivalry exists between the two hypotheses and the final outcome is unlikely to be based only on regional and species differences. Even studies on the same tissue from the same species provide contradictory data and make conclusive statements difficult to make.

GANGLIONIC TRANSMISSION

Intramural ganglia

Although a variety of transmitter substances have so far been discussed which directly affect muscle contractility, by far the greatest proportion of potential neurotransmitters can be found within the enteric nervous system (Table 4.1).

Acetylcholine (ACh) is the major parasympathetic preganglionic transmitter acting through nicotinic receptors to cause postsynaptic depolarization. However, it has also been suggested that 5-HT is involved in ganglionic transmission in the inhibitory parasympathetic pathway. Noradrenaline is the postganglionic sympathetic transmitter which, from its

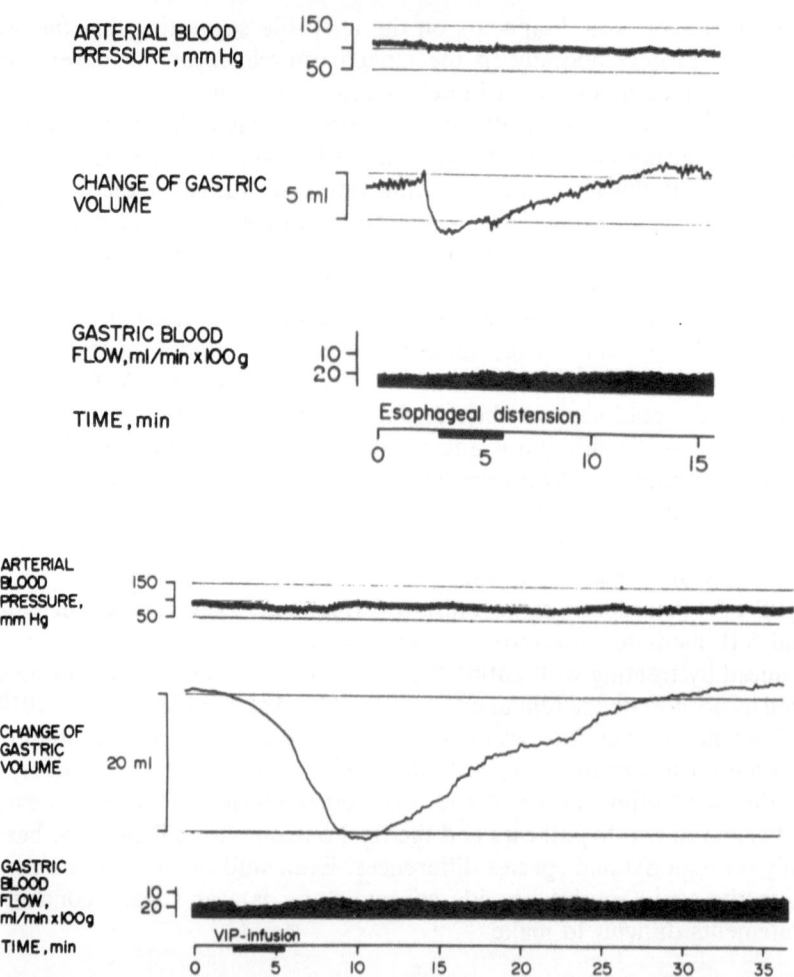

Figure 4.6 Comparison of nerve-mediated and VIP mediated relaxations of the cat stomach. Relaxation of the stomach is reflected as a downward deflection of the gastric volume recording. Upper record: reflex relaxation elicited by oesophageal distension. Lower record: the response to a close arterial infusion of VIP at a rate of $3.4\,nmol\,min^{-1}$ (From Eklund *et al.*, 1979, with kind permission of the authors and the editor of Acta Physiol. Scand.)

histochemical detection in the intramural ganglia and not in the muscle layer, is suggested to have a primarily ganglionic action.

Mamber and Gershon (1979) investigated the relationship between the sympathetic nerves and the enteric ganglia by measuring the output of tritiated ACh from intestinal segments as a measure of ganglionic transmission. Transmural stimulation increased this ACh output but during simultaneous stimulation of the sympathetic nerves the output was inhibited. The inhibitory effect of sympathetic stimulation was prevented by pretreating the animals with 6-hydroxydopamine to deplete the noradrenaline stored in

Table 4.1 Substances located within neural elements of the enteric ganglia, the evidence for some of these playing a transmitter role is somewhat equivocal. Note that many of these substances have hormonal roles elsewhere in the body

Acetylcholine (ACh)
5-Hydroxytryptamine (5-HT)
Dopamine
Noradrenaline
Adenosine triphosphate (ATP)
Gamma-aminobutyric acid (GABA)
SubstanceP
Vasoactive intestinal polypeptide (VIP)
Enkephalin
Somatostatin
Pancreatic polypeptide (PP)
Angiotensin
Adrenocorticotrophic hormone (ACTH)
Cholecystokinin (CCK)
Bombesin
Neurotensin

sympathetic nerve endings. Thus release of noradrenaline from sympathetic nerves reduces the output of ACh from the intramural ganglia. The output of tritiated noradrenaline was similarly inhibited by ACh. Atropine enhanced the release of noradrenaline suggesting that tonic activity in cholinergic nerves was inhibiting the action of the sympathetic nerves. Ultrastructural observations indicated that noradrenergic and cholinergic terminals were in close proximity and could, therefore, influence each other via axoaxonic synapses. Thus, the action of sympathetic nerves would be suppressed while the parasympathetic nerves were active, while activation of the sympathetic nerves would inhibit the release of acetylcholine. This presynaptic modulation would sharpen the effect of excitatory and inhibitory reflexes by reducing the output of an antagonist transmitter.

In sphincters, the action of the sympathetic nerves is generally the opposite of that seen elsewhere in the gastrointestinal tract. In the lower oesophageal sphincter, for example, noradrenaline depolarizes the smooth muscle cells resulting in contraction and an increase in sphincter tone. The effect is antagonized by atropine because the noradrenaline, via alpha-adrenoreceptors, potentiates the release of ACh from cholinergic terminals (see p. 88). Thus, irrespective of whether sympathetic nerves cause contraction or relaxation of gastrointestinal smooth muscle, noradrenaline acts in part by modifying the cholinergic pathway to the muscle.

The recording of neuronal activity in the enteric nervous system and the effect of iontophoretic application of putative transmitters on this activity is a method of assessing directly potential transmitter action. ACh has an excitatory effect on both S-type neurones recorded intracellularly and the extracellularly recorded single spike neurones (see Chapter 2). These effects are mediated through nicotinic receptors typical of ganglionic transmission and resemble the fast excitatory postsynaptic potentials recorded spontaneously. From the blocking effect of hexamethonium (a nicotinic receptor antagonist) on spontaneous excitatory postsynaptic potentials and on ganglionic transmission following stimulation of the interganglionic nerve bundles and preganglionic parasympathetic stimulation it is apparent that ACh is the major interneuronal transmitter in the enteric plexuses. The amplitude of the fast excitatory postsynaptic potential is reduced by noradrenaline supporting the view that noradrenergic action is mediated through presynaptic inhibition of the release of ACh. Many other substances including 5-HT, ATP, somatostatin and enkephalin may also have actions via presynaptic modulation of transmitter release. Enkephalin is especially abundant in the myenteric plexus and is present in about one-quarter of S-type cells (Bornstein et al., 1984). This density of enkephalin-immunoreactive neurones would imply an important role for enkephalin in ganglionic transmission and undoubtedly contribute to the gastrointestinal motor disturbances that are a side-effect of morphine use.

The transmitter responsible for the slow excitatory postsynaptic potential seen in the AH cells (p. 27) has also received detailed consideration and two candidates exist at present. Wood (1981) suggests 5-HT following his report of mimickry between iontophoretic application of 5-HT and nerve-mediated slow excitatory postsynaptic potentials. Tachyphylaxis to 5-HT application is paralleled by a reduction in nerve-mediated response. Morita, Katayama and North (1980), on the other hand, find that the response to nerve stimulation can be reduced by treatment with chymotrypsin while the response to 5-HT remains unchanged. Any peptide released by nerve stimulation would be destroyed by this powerful proteolytic enzyme, provided that it gained access to the the site of transmitter release within the ganglia, and since the effect of iontophoretically applied substance P is similarly reduced might indicate that a peptide, and possibly substance P, was the transmitter. The transmitter for the slow inhibitory postsynaptic potential is considered to be a catecholamine, possibly dopamine, but this area has not been systematically studied.

Different populations of neurones show different responses to individual putative transmitters, some depolarized, some hyperpolarized, and some having no effect. There is therefore a degree of biological specificity suggesting a physiological role for these substances in ganglionic transmission. Recent studies indicate that some neurones release more than one transmitter (Burnstock, 1981; Hokfelt et al., 1980). ATP is released along with ACh and noradrenaline where it may act prejunctionally to modify transmitter output. Peptides have also been demonstrated to coexist with more conventional transmitters. Thus somatostatin has been identified in some noradrenergic nerves, VIP has been found along with ACh and substance P in 5-HT-containing neurones. These peptides may act as co-transmitters, both having postsynaptic actions; alternatively they may act as neuromodulators that modify the release or action of the conventional transmitters.

Prevertebral ganglia

The organization of the prevertebral ganglia (see p. 48) is far more complex than a simple relay station for the sympathetic nerves destined for the abdominal viscera. They are integrative centres receiving a sensory input from peripheral sources in addition to the preganglionic sympathetic connection from the spinal cord. Both slow and fast synaptic processes determine the level of neuronal traffic in the postganglionic noradrenergic nerves innervating the gastrointestinal tract.

Individual ganglion cells receive a cholinergic preganglionic input, the released ACh acting on nicotinic receptors to generate a fast excitatory postsynaptic potential in a similar way to that described in the intramural ganglia. The integrative interactions between individual excitatory postsynaptic potentials is achieved by convergence of presynaptic inputs from different sources. In the inferior mesenteric ganglia, for example, individual ganglion cells are excited by stimulation of any of the different nerve bundles connecting it with adjacent viscera, ganglia and the spinal cord (Szurszewski, 1977a). Divergence of the presynaptic input also occurs with individual fibres branching to innervate several ganglion cells. Thus temporal and spatial summation of individual postsynaptic potentials determine the final outflow to the gut. An additional slow synaptic potential giving rise to excitatory membrane events lasting many seconds extends the integrative function, since it can convert a subthreshold fast excitatory postsynaptic potential into an action potential that will propagate to the target of the postganglionic cell. In the guinea-pig, the prevertebral ganglia contain a network of fibres which show immunoreactivity to a number of peptides including VIP, somatostatin, enkephalin and substanceP.

GASTROINTESTINAL HORMONES

A physiological role for many of the putative gastrointestinal hormones has not yet been established (see Walsh, 1981; Bertaccini, 1982). Only gastrin, CCK, secretin, and glucose-dependent insulinotropic peptide (GIP) can be considered as true hormones with any degree of confidence and the primary actions of all of these (except CCK) are on secretory processes within the gastrointestinal tract. Motility changes mediated via hormones are evident from responses noted in totally denervated or auto-transplanted regions of gut. However, the actual hormone(s) responsible can only be speculated upon from knowledge of the effect of intravenous infusion of exogenous hormone at levels similar to those found in the blood following a meal.

With the recent developments in protein chemistry and the discovery of very many more peptides (Table 4.2) in the epithelial lining of the gastrointestinal tract the concept of the gut mucosa as a diffuse endocrine organ has arisen. These peptides appear to have roles relevant to different aspects of secretion, absorption, gut development and growth as well as to the control of motility. The evidence for the latter is considered in Chapters 5 to 10 dealing with regional aspects of fed and fasted motility. Here, I merely want to raise the concept of the gut as an endocrine organ.

Table 4.2 Gastrointestinal hormones: substances located within the epithelial lining of the gastrointestinal tract. The major site of cells containing these peptides and the main intraluminal stimuli causing their release is also shown. Note that some have already been considered as neurotransmitters. Duo = duodenum; jej = jejunum

Hormone	Distribution	Released by
Gastrin	Antrum	Peptides
CCK-PZ	Duo/jej	Fatty acids
Secretin	Duo/jej	Acid
GIP	Duo/jej	Glucose
Enteroglucagon	Ileum/colon	Fats
Motilin	Duo/jej	Nutrients (inhibit)
Pancreatic polypeptide (PP)	Pancreas	Peptides
Neurotensin	Ileum	Fats
Gastrin-releasing polypeptide	Stomach	Nutrients
Somatostatin	Stomach/intestine	Nutrients
Enkephalin	Duo	

Some of the examples in Table 4.2 are considered to serve a more paracrine function. The location of somatostatin-like immunity in cells closely associated with gastrin and CCK-containing cells, and also within the islets of Langerhans, suggests that somatostatin may be involved in the regulation of the release of other hormones into the bloodstream. Enroute to the blood capillaries hormones may cause local effects in adjacent cells. It is difficult, therefore, to separate the gut hormones into functional classes where some have only local effects while others mediate their controlling influence after passage through the circulation. Other hormones may be released by nervous action.

Endocrine–paracrine cells are found in the epithelial lining scattered diffusely along the whole length of the gastrointestinal tract and have been classified on the basis of their cellular content. Although differences occur between these different cell types they all have essential similarities (Figure 4.7). The surface of the cell in contact with the lumen of the gut has microvilli which, it is postulated, act as a receptor sensing luminal contents for pH or levels of various nutrients. The secretory granules of hormone are contained within vesicles and stored at the base of the cell ready for release into the interstitial space.

Many of the hormones exist in multiple forms with different chain

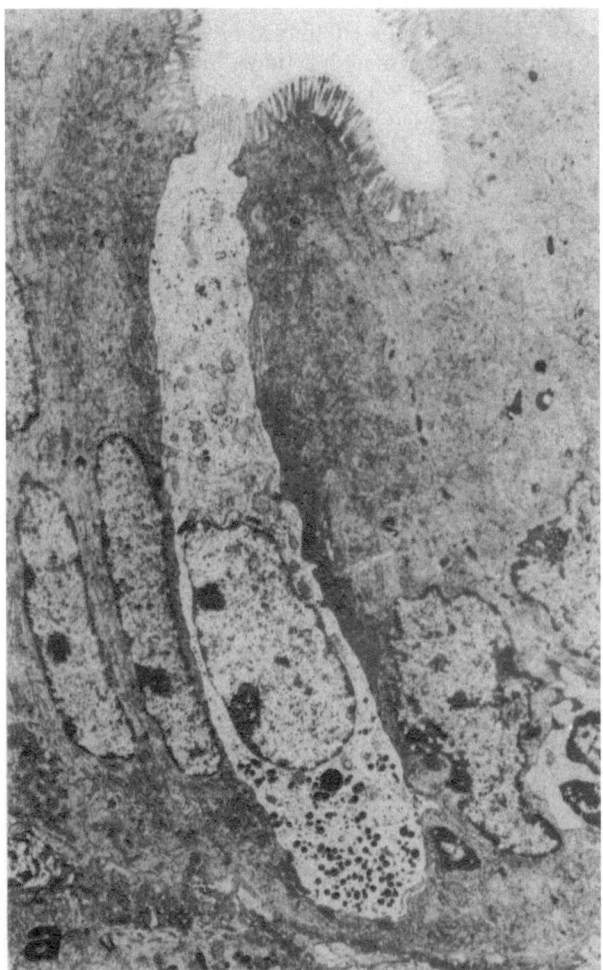

Figure 4.7 S (secretin containing) cell of the human jejunum. Magnification 3160×. The cell extends from the lumen to just above the basal membrane of the epithelium. The luminal end shows a tuft of microvilli which is slightly different from the adjacent absorptive cells. The basal part of the cell contains vesicles of secretory granules (From Solcia *et al.*, 1981, with kind permission of the author and publisher, Raven Press)

lengths, different half-lives and different potencies. The C-terminal octa-peptide of CCK (CCK-8) has been mentioned as the main form of CCK found stored and released from nerve terminals. This peptide together with an N-terminal-extended CCK-33 are released into the portal blood following a meal. Larger forms have been described with further N-terminal extensions, for example, CCK-39, while bigger versions still are considered as the prohormone. The same is true for gastrin with G-17 and G-34 as the main hormonal forms. The sequence of the C-terminal –four amino acids of CCK and gastrin are identical giving rise to similarities of action of these two hormones. This smaller version of CCK/gastrin has been suggested as another form which may have biological actions in the nervous system. Other hormones have similarities in aminoacid sequence and overlap in biological actions; thus, the secretin family of peptides contain VIP, glucagon and GIP.

A common question asked is why are there so many of these 'gut peptides'? One explanation is probably as a consequence of their many different roles as regulators of secretion, absorption, motility, and development and growth. Another reason is starting to emerge from research by molecular biologists addressing the problem of DNA transcription and translation during synthesis of individual gut peptides. They find sequences of DNA representing the preprohormone which has peptide chains removed from both C- and N-terminals before the 'final' hormone is packaged ready for release. Within these much larger structures are sequences of amino acids corresponding to other peptides. It may turn out then that multiple hormones are derived from the same precursor. New peptides and peptide fragments are constantly being identified in the gastrointestinal tract, but what still needs to be established is their physiological significance.

5
The oesophagus

INTRODUCTION

The oesophagus is a long narrow muscular tube which in man is approximately 25 cm long. It connects the pharynx with the stomach providing a
conduit for bidirectional flow. Ingested material is actively propelled into
the stomach by means of peristaltic contractions that are initiated by
swallowing or when a bolus of food becomes lodged in the oesophagus.
However, during vomiting the reverse occurs, but under these circumstances the force propelling gastric contents into the mouth is not derived
from oesophageal peristalsis but from contractions of the abdominal
muscles and diaphragm. At rest the oesophagus is closed by sphincters at
both ends. The upper oesophageal sphincter is constricted so that air is
prevented from entering the oseophagus during inspiration while tone in
the lower oesophageal sphincter minimizes the reflux of acidic gastric
contents.

   The proximal third of the oesophagus is composed of longitudinally and
circularly orientated striated muscle and as such is totally dependent on
its extrinsic nerve supply from the vagus nerve. The distal third and lower
oesophageal sphincter is composed entirely of smooth muscle which is
continuous with the corresponding layers of striated muscle. However,
unlike the smooth muscle in the stomach and intestine, oesophageal smooth
muscle does not show phasic slow wave activity and is highly dependent
on its nerve supply from both extrinsic and intrinsic sources. The mid-
oesophageal region is the transition zone where striated muscle gradually
gives way to smooth muscle. The striated and smooth muscle regions are
subjected to different controls, yet the peristaltic waves initiated in the
striated portion propagate smoothly through the transition zone and on
towards the stomach. In this chapter the current concepts of the mechanisms
regulating and coordinating the different portions of oesophagus are discussed.

OESOPHAGEAL PERISTALSIS

The relative accessibility of the oesophagus has enabled the sequence of events associated with oesophageal peristalsis to be fully characterized. Radiographic studies during the swallowing of contrast medium have been used in the past to visualize the passage of fluid from the mouth into the stomach. Manometric recordings of pressure profiles in the oesophagus allow quantification of the peristaltic wave in terms of force and duration of contraction. At rest the oesophagus is flaccid and intraluminal pressure approximates that of the intrapleural pressure and consequently varies with the respiratory cycle, being more negative during inspiration. Oesophageal peristalsis is usually initiated by swallowing. This can be done voluntarily but as the bolus of food enters the pharynx it becomes an involuntary action and is reflexly activated as a consequence of stimulation of receptors in the palate, pharynx and epiglottis. In anaesthetized animals the swallowing (deglutition) reflex can be evoked by electrical stimulation of the afferent fibres innervating this region, especially those in the superior laryngeal branch of the vagus nerves. The buccal and pharyngeal phases of swallowing direct the bolus of food towards the oesophagus by the sequential contraction of a number of pharyngeal muscle groups. At the same time there is closure of the nasal and tracheal passages to prevent the bolus deviating from its required path and opening of the upper oesophageal sphincter during which time the bolus enters the oesophagus. The pressure in the upper oesophageal sphincter, maintained between 100 and 130 mmHg at rest, falls briefly to atmospheric pressure as a consequence of relaxation of the cricopharyngeus muscle and a forward displacement of the larynx. The pharyngeal phase ends with pressure in the upper oesophageal sphincter rising above resting levels for a few seconds before finally returning to its resting tone.

Oesophageal peristalsis begins just below the upper oesophageal sphincter just as the sphincter is closing and sweeps caudally at between 2 and 5 cm s^{-1} taking about 6 s to reach the stomach. As the peristaltic wave passes over a stationary catheter positioned in the oesophagus the pressure generated by the contraction can be recorded as a transient rise and fall in pressure which lasts between 2 and 4 s and reaches a maximum pressure of approximately 75 mmHg. A series of such catheters records the smooth progression of the wave as it passes from the striated to the smooth muscle portion and approaches the stomach (Figure 5.1). The lower oesophageal sphincter, which at rest is closed, begins to open as oesophageal peristalsis develops and remains open until the bolus has finally reached the stomach, although with repeated swallowing it may remain open for longer.

Should a bolus become lodged in the oesophagus, a reflex is activated which elicits 'secondary peristalsis'. These waves of contraction occur without any swallowing movements or without conscious awareness and

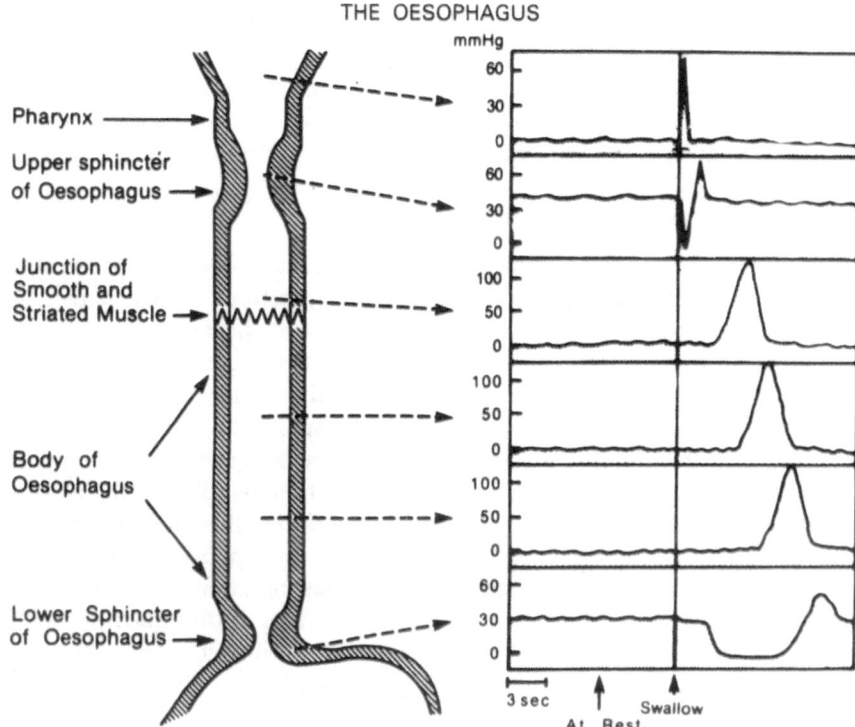

Figure 5.1 Sequence in time of pressure changes in the oesophageal sphincters and body during swallowing (From Christensen, 1983, with kind permission of the author and publisher, Wright, PSG)

start above the bolus, sweeping down repeatedly until the bolus has been removed. This phenomenon illustrates the importance of the sensory innervation of the oesophagus which also plays a part in the progression of the 'primary' peristaltic waves elicited by swallowing.

CONTROL OF OESOPHAGEAL MOTILITY

The striated muscle portion

While oesophageal peristalsis has been well characterized in man, any description of the controlling influences has depended upon the use of a suitable animal model. For studies of the striated muscle portion the dog, rabbit, guinea-pig, rat and sheep have been widely employed, because in these animals the whole oesophagus as far as the lower oesophageal sphincter consists of striated muscle.

Striated muscle throughout the body is controlled by neurogenic mechanisms, that is they contract only when nerve impulses pass along their motor nerves and release acetylcholine from their endplates. One might logically argue, therefore, that contractions of the upper oesophageal sphincter depend on continuous discharge in the nerves innervating this region, while the peristaltic wave in the oesophagus occurs as a consequence of sequential activation of progressively caudal segments of the oesophagus.

The upper oesophageal sphincter

Closure of the upper oesophageal sphincter is maintained by contractions of the muscles surrounding the pharyngeal junction. In man and dog, electromyographic (emg) recordings from muscles in this region indicate continuous tonic activity in the cricopharyngeus muscle which flattens the oesophagus against the cricoid cartilage. This results in an asymmetric pressure profile in the upper oesophageal sphincter with the pressure recorded in the anterior and posterior direction being considerably higher than that laterally. During deglutition the continuous spiking emg activity is immediately and completely inhibited, and during this time the pressure in the upper oesophageal sphincter falls. As the sphincter closes again there is an intense burst of spiking activity lasting about a second which then subsides to resting levels. Since emg activity in the muscle exactly matches the spincter tone it seems reasonable to conclude that contractile activity in the cricopharyngeus keeps the upper oesophageal sphincter closed, while relaxation is associated with suppression of the muscle's contractile activity.

The motor innervation to the upper oesophageal region is from the superior laryngeal nerve. Electrophysiological recordings from this nerve reveal a population of efferent fibres whose discharge correlates precisely with that of the cricopharyngeus muscle, that is they carry a tonic discharge which is briefly interrupted during the pharyngeal phase of a swallow (Andrews, 1956). Relaxation of the upper oesophageal sphincter is therefore due to central inhibition of the motor innervation rather than to activation of an inhibitory nerve supply. A slight pressure of about 10mmHg, however, still exists after the motor nerves to the upper oesophageal sphincter have been sectioned. This residual pressure falls to zero during deglutition as a consequence of the forward and upward movement of the larynx brought about by contraction of the suprahyoid muscles. The cricopharyngeus muscle relaxes but sphincter opening is due to contraction of the suprahyoid muscles.

The oesophageal body

Three pieces of evidence confirm the neurogenic mechanisms of the striated portion of the oesophagus. First, vagotomy, above the level where the vagus nerves branch to innervate the oesophagus, or nicotinic cholinoreceptor blockade abolish oesophageal peristalsis. Second, electrical stimulation of the motor innervation leads to the simultaneous contraction of the whole striated muscle portion indicating that under normal circumstances progressively distal segments are activated in sequence. This is borne out finally by the observation that transection of the oesophagus does not prevent the caudal progression of the primary peristaltic wave; the contractions can jump the gap created by the transection. In primary peristalsis, therefore, there is no requirement for the presence of a bolus in the oesophagus. The peristaltic contractions are programmed centrally and once initiated run from beginning to end without any further afferent input. However, there is an extensive sensory innervation with mechanoreceptors in the wall of the oesophagus detecting the presence of a bolus or contraction of the muscle. Recent evidence suggests that these afferent fibres may also contribute to primary peristalsis. In the sheep the sensory innervation to the thoracic oesophagus can be removed totally by complete vagal section on one side combined with section of the nodose ganglion on the other side, the efferent supply from this side being kept intact (Falempin and Rousseau, 1984). After this procedure primary peristaltic waves do not extend into the deafferented segment and secondary peristalsis is abolished. Thus afferent signals must reinforce the central mechanism and allow the force and progression of the peristaltic wave to be adjusted according to both oesophageal contents and its contractions. The afferent information is conducted rapidly to the brainstem via small myelinated nerve fibres and provides the afferent limb for secondary peristalsis initiated by oesophageal distension, where a peristaltic wave of contraction occurs without prior contraction of the pharyngeal muscles.

Thus there is a central programme which is continuously modified by sensory feedback to provide a motor sequence which progressively activates muscles of the pharynx and oesophagus directing the bolus of food towards the stomach. Specific lesions in the CNS indicate that the circuitry generating this programme lies in the brainstem. The motor outflow to the striated muscle originates in the nucleus ambiguus while the smooth muscle portion receives its supply from the dorsal motor nucleus. In both cases the pathway to the oesophagus is in the vagus nerves. The activity of the vagal efferent fibres innervating the various levels of oesophagus have been investigated by recording directly from the vagus nerve (Andrews, 1956), and by the nerve suture technique described in Chapter 3. In the latter, the central end of the left vagus nerve was sutured to the peripheral end of the spinal accessory nerve innervating the sternomastoid muscles. Following reinnervation contractions of muscle fibres (recorded with emg electrodes) represent the discharge of their new vagal innervation. The vagal motor fibres had no spontaneous impulse traffic, but generated a burst of action potentials during both primary and secondary oesophageal peristalsis with the former generating a more powerful burst of action potentials (Roman and Tieffenbach, 1972). Different motor fibres discharged action potentials at different times during the propagated peristaltic wave indicating that they were activated in turn to produce a craniocaudal sequence of oesophageal contraction. Afferent inputs reinforced the vagal motor discharge since a more powerful discharge was recorded when a bolus was present in the oesophagus. This afferent input to the brainstem is by way of the nucleus of the tractus solitarius. Between this region and the site of the motor outflow lies the integrative circuitry which organizes the successive excitation of motor neurones. Electrical stimulation of this region readily evokes the swallowing sequence while microelectrode recordings in this region detect neurones activated during swallowing or whose spontaneous discharge is altered during swallowing. Again from the temporal relationship with oesophageal activity it would seem that these neurones are involved in the generation of the motor sequence. The discharge in these neurones continues in animals treated with curare to block oesophageal contractions and so is not dependent upon the input from afferent fibres activated during contraction or passage of a bolus. Inhibitory phenomena have also been described in those interneurones involved in the regulation of motor discharge to more distal oesophageal regions and are suggested to be responsible for the inhibition of distal motor neurones during contractions of the proximal oesophagus.

The central mechanisms associated with secondary peristalsis are not very different from those for primary peristalsis. The motorneurones and interneurones are the same but excitation is weaker during secondary peristalsis and does not involve the contraction of pharyngeal muscles. This lower level of neuronal excitability observed during secondary peristalsis is enhanced by afferent inputs from oesophageal mechanoreceptors without which the central programme fails to reach threshold. Thus secondary peristaltic waves cannot jump a gap provided by oesophageal transection.

The smooth muscle portion

The study of the mechanisms controlling the smooth muscle portion of the oesophagus have again depended on suitable animal models. The experimental details outlined below are from studies of oesophageal peristalsis in primates, cat and more recently in the North American opossum, animals whose distal oesophagus is, like man, composed of smooth muscle.

The differences in controlling mechanisms associated with the striated and smooth muscle portions are dramatically illustrated by the effect of vagotomy which totally paralyses the striated muscle but not the smooth muscle portion. In vagotomized animals, or even totally isolated segments of distal oesophagus, the inflation of a small balloon within the lumen elicits peristaltic contractions which sweep caudally. Similarly, in contrast to the striated muscle oesophagus, electrical stimulation of the peripheral ends of the sectioned vagus nerves evokes propagating waves of contraction.

It would appear therefore that a peripheral mechanism controls the peristaltic waves in the distal oesophagus.

During normal swallowing the peristaltic wave passes smoothly from the striated portion through the transition zone and into the smooth muscle section without any sign of interruption. This may represent activation of the distal oesophagus as part of the centrally determined craniocaudal sequence. Alternatively, since balloon distension can evoke peristalsis in the distal portion without central involvement, it is possible that the arrival of a bolus of food into the smooth muscle region during a normal swallow provides the stimulus for continued peristalsis. This possibility can be tested by preventing the arrival of the bolus. Oesophagostomy in the cervical oesophagus to divert the bolus to the outside does not prevent thoracic oesophageal peristalsis. Also, treatment with curare, which blocks nicotinic cholinoreceptors on the striated muscle, prevents striated muscle contractions and thus blocks the propulsion of a bolus into the smooth muscle portion but does not eliminate the distal peristaltic wave. A central command would therefore appear to initiate peristalsis in the distal oesophagus but, once initiated, peristalsis can proceed without further central support.

Recent investigations of distal oesophageal peristalsis have concentrated on attempts to elucidate the peripheral control mechanisms. Two possible sites for control exist. The peristalsis could be a myogenic property of the smooth muscle itself or could depend on control by the intramural plexuses.

Electrical stimuli applied either to the vagal innervation or directly to the wall of the oesophagus (transmural stimulation) elicit a complex contractile response which in the circular muscle layer has essentially two components (Figure 5.2). The first, called the 'on' or 'early' response, begins soon after the onset of stimulation and propagates caudally along the oesophagus; this response is blocked by atropinization and is therefore due to excitation of cholinergic intramural nerves (Dodds et al., 1978). The second component occurs after the stimulation has ceased and is termed the 'off' or 'rebound' contraction; this too propagates caudally but at a velocity faster than that seen for the 'on' response or normal peristalsis. The 'off' response is associated with prior hyperpolarization of the smooth muscle cell membrane during the period of stimulation. However, without tone in the oesophagus this hyperpolarization does not result in actual relaxation of the muscle. Instead, a 'rebound' contraction follows removal of the stimulus as the membrane potential rises to a level above threshold for the generation of spike potentials and contraction. The hyperpolarization is the result of release of an inhibitory transmitter which falls in the class of non-adrenergic, non-cholinergic transmitters discussed in Chapter 4. There is considerable speculation as to whether the 'rebound' contraction is the direct result of the preceding hyperpolarization, or whether a second excitatory non-adrenergic, non-cholinergic transmitter is simultaneously released, but whose depolarizing effect is only seen as the effect of the inhibitory transmitter wears off.

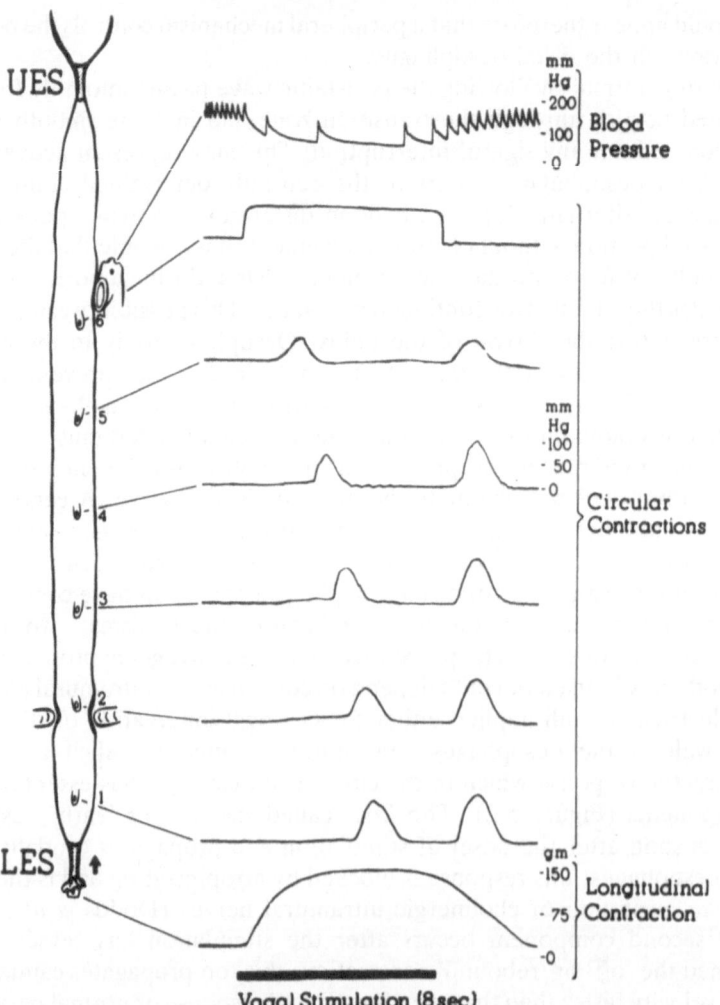

UES

mm
Hg
- 200
- 100
- 0

Blood
Pressure

mm
Hg
-100
- 50
-0

Circular
Contractions

LES

gm
-150
- 75
-0

Longitudinal
Contraction

Vagal Stimulation (8 sec)

Figure 5.2 Circular and longitudinal muscle contractions in the oesophagus of the opossum elicited by cervical vagal stimulation of 8 s duration. 'On' and 'off' contractions are evident in the circular muscle layer of the smooth muscle portion (manometric sites 5–1). A square-shaped, striated muscle contraction was recorded at the level of the aortic arch (site 6) and a sustained contraction of the longitudinal muscle was also elicited. Cardiac slowing marks the duration of the stimulation (From Dodds *et al.*, 1981, with kind permission of the author and the editor of Am. J. Physiol.)

The question that has to be addressed now is how do the responses to electrical stimulation relate to oesophageal peristalsis seen during swallowing? In terms of velocity of propagation the 'on' response more closely matches that seen during peristalsis although the velocity can vary depending on the stimulation parameters. However, if the 'on' response represents normal peristalsis one would expect the latter to be abolished by muscarinic cholinergic blockade with, for example, atropine. This is not the case and so points towards a 'rebound' phenomenon.

Weisbrodt and Christensen (1972) put forward the hypothesis that peristalsis was a 'rebound' contraction which propagated at a velocity determined by the latency gradient for development of a 'rebound' response.

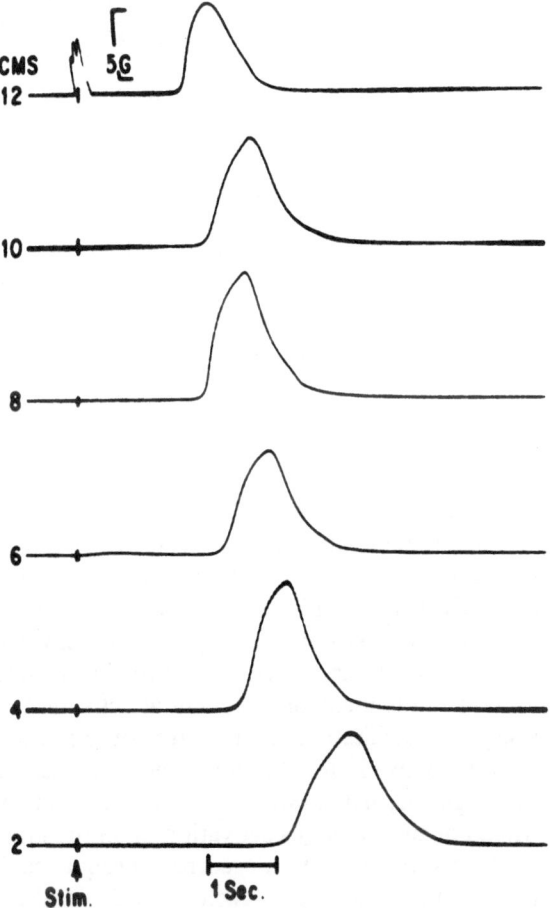

Figure 5.3 Response of isolated strips of circular smooth muscle from different levels of opossum oesophagus to transmural stimulation (at arrow). Distance is in centimeters from gastro-oesophageal junction (From Weisbrodt and Christensen, 1972, with kind permission of the authors and the editor of Gastroenterology)

Figure 5.3 illustrates the experiments leading to this hypothesis. Isolated strips of smooth muscle from progressively distal regions of the opossum oesophagus were maintained separately *in vitro*. When stimulated transmurally, the rebound that followed the end of a train of stimuli occurred after a latency which became progressively longer with more distal segments. Had these individual strips of oesophagus been connected, the velocity of propagation calculated from their latencies correlated with that shown for the 'rebound' response seen in the intact oesophagus.

The source of this latency gradient may be within the muscle itself or could depend on the rate of release and inactivation of a neurotransmitter. Smooth muscle from progressively distal segments shows a gradient in internal potassium ion concentration being lower in more distal regions with a corresponding gradient in resting menbrane potential. The increase in latency distally may be a function of these gradients and could be accounted for by differences in membrane permeability to potassium ions following hyperpolarization (Christensen, 1983).

Thus, according to the rebound theory, the output from the central programme to the oesophageal smooth muscle is one of simultaneous activation of the inhibitory innervation. As the peristaltic wave nears the end of the striated portion nervous activity in the inhibitory pathway ceases allowing a 'rebound' contraction to develop in the most proximal smooth muscle region which then sweeps down the remainder of the oesophagus. Such a mechanism would depend on accurate timing of the termination of the vagal efferent discharge to allow a 'rebound' contraction to take over smoothly from the striated muscle contractions. Additionally, the central and peripheral mechanisms must be matched so that the velocity of propagation in the two oesophageal regions are similar.

The patterns of neuronal firing in efferent fibres destined for the distal oesophagus are not consistent with this hypothesis. In Roman and Tieffen-bach's (1972) studies on the conscious monkey the vagal efferent discharge was recorded indirectly using the nerve suture technique. The vagal fibres generated a burst of a few spikes at low frequency which were temporally related to primary and secondary peristaltic waves in the smooth muscle portion with different fibres indicating sequential activation. This type of activity was envisaged as facilitating the discharge of excitatory intramural neurones that were responsible for the organized sequence of peristalsis. Such a pattern of vagal discharge could, however, also fit the 'rebound' hypothesis if, instead of simultaneous activation of all the inhibitory nerve fibres to the oesophagus, the activation occurred in sequence. Under these circumstances the timing of the end of each burst of vagal activity at the different oesophageal levels would determine the propagated sequence. Such a mechanism could also delay the velocity of propagation of the 'rebound' to that seen during swallowing.

Since balloon distension can elicit peristalsis *in vitro*, the intramural plexuses must contain all the elements of a reflex arc. Under these circumstances, oesophageal peristalsis is associated with inhibition distally and contraction orally in a way reminiscent of peristalsis in the intestine (see Chapter 2). This parallel with the small intestine led Diamant and El-Sharkawy, (1977) to propose a model for oesophageal peristalsis based on a series of local circuits in the enteric nervous system which coordinate contractions in the longitudinal and circular muscle layers with prior descending inhibition of the circular muscle layer. Activation of these circuits by either local reflexes or following extrinsic input as part of the central programme for swallowing would account for peristalsis seen *in vivo* and *in vitro*. In this hypothesis contractions depend on both cholinergic and non-cholinergic transmitters with the former playing a permissive role since atropine does not prevent oesophageal peristalsis. By analogy with the small intestine, oesophageal contractions may also involve disinhibition of a tonic inhibitory innervation. The velocity of propagation would be determined by the sequential synaptic delays along the oesophagus.

Of these two hypotheses I favour the latter for two reasons. Firstly, because rebound contractions are a phenomenon associated with the abrupt cessation of bursts of electrical stimulation applied to non-adrenergic, non-cholinergic inhibitory nerves. Manipulating the train of electrical impulses so that the stimulus frequency wanes rather than stops abruptly results in the marked attenuation of rebound contractions (Andrews and Grundy, 1981). While the motor innervation to the oesophagus does generate discrete bursts of impulses during both primary and secondary peristalsis these bursts are of low frequency and do not end abruptly but show a gradual decline in frequency. Rebound contractions may, therefore, be an artifact of electrical stimulation rather than a functional mechanism for generating contractions.

Secondly, it seems a roundabout way of producing propagated waves of contraction. It is easier to visualize a controlled contraction being the direct result of a change in neuronal firing, be it enhanced activity in excitatory nerves or the suppression of an inhibitory innervation. In both cases the resulting contraction occurs during the change in discharge and so can be subjected to feedback regulation from receptors detecting the passage of the wave of contraction. A rebound contraction, because it follows the end of the stimulus, would, once initiated, be out of control.

The lower oesophageal sphincter

The lower oesophageal sphincter is one of the most intensely studied regions of the gastrointestinal tract. This is partly because of its complex and still controversial control mechanisms and partly because of clinical interest in the aetiology of gastro-oesophageal reflux.

Controversy arose initially over the actual existence of a sphincter between the oesophagus and stomach. Anatomically smooth muscle in this region is no different from that on either side with regard to thickness of muscle layers or morphology of smooth muscle cells. However, functionally a region of high pressure exists around the point where the oesophagus passes through the diaphragm. This high pressure zone can be demonstrated manometrically using a 'pull-through technique', a method which measures

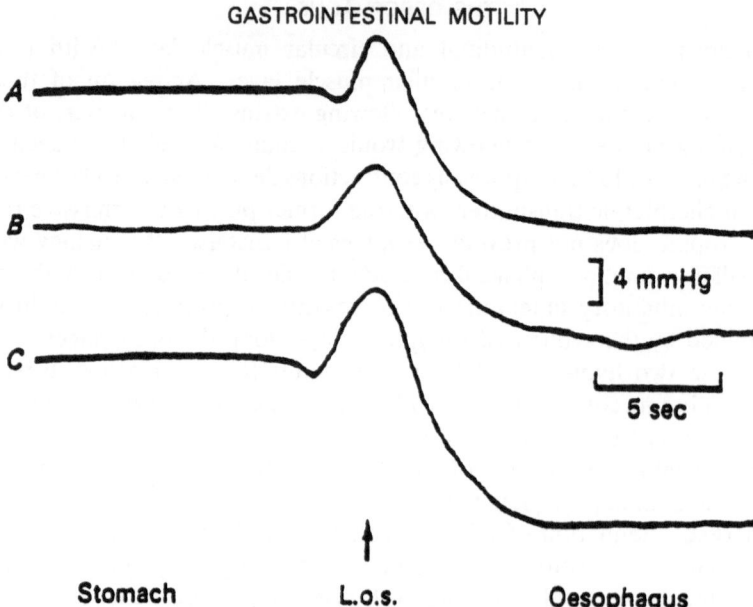

A

B

] 4 mmHg

C

|_____| 5 sec

↑

Stomach　　　　**L.o.s.**　　　　**Oesophagus**

Figure 5.4 Pressure profile, observed in anaesthetized cats, during the withdrawal of an open tip catheter from stomach to oesophagus. Each tracing comes from a different animal. The high pressure zone corresponds to the lower oesophageal sphincter (l.o.s.). The pressure is higher in the stomach than oesophagus (From Gonella, Niel and Roman, 1977, with kind permission of the authors and the editor of J. Physiol. (London))

the pressure from the end of a catheter as it is withdrawn at constant speed from the stomach into the oesophagus (Figure 5.4). In man the length of the high-pressure zone, calculated from the pressure profile, varies between 2 and 4 cm with a peak pressure maintaining closure of about 20 mmHg generated by tonic contraction of the circular muscle layer. This pressure, however, can vary considerably especially during swallowing when the high pressure zone disappears to allow the passage of a bolus into the stomach.

The question of active sphincter relaxation during swallowing was considered for some time to be an artifact of measuring sphincter pressure with a stationary catheter positioned in the region of the lower oesophageal sphincter. During swallowing, contraction of the longitudinal muscle layer results in a significant reduction in the total length of the oesophagus. A stationary catheter would consequently be displaced from the lower oesophageal sphincter and move transiently into the stomach where a lower basal pressure exists. However, a rapid 'pull through' during the oesophageal phase of swallowing fails to detect a high pressure zone indicating that relaxation of the sphincter has occurred. The relaxation is not considered to open the sphincter but to reduce tone sufficiently to allow the bolus to pass through as it is propelled forward by the advancing peristaltic wave.

Relaxation of the lower oesophageal sphincter starts early during the swallowing reflex, the pressure falling as the wave of peristalsis passes along the cervical portion of the oesophagus. The relaxation continues for between 5 and 10 s and is followed by a pressure rise above basal levels for a period of approximately the same duration. This aftercontraction is in peristaltic continuity with the oesophageal contraction, and so firmly closes the sphincter after the bolus has passed into the stomach. With repeated swallows the sphincter may remain open throughout until the peristaltic wave associated with the last swallow has passed. In man, swallowed fluids fall rapidly under gravity ahead of the wave of contraction and may arrive at the lower oesophageal sphincter before it has relaxed, so its entry into the stomach is held up until relaxation occurs.

Research into the functioning of the lower oesophageal sphincter has followed two distinct lines: the mechanisms responsible for generating the basal sphincter tone, and those mediating relaxation of the sphincter. In both types of study complications arise because of species differences between those animals with striated muscle and those with smooth muscle in the terminal oesophagus.

Sphincter tone

The high pressure zone is generated by high tone in the circular muscle layer. This is partly due to myogenic properties and partly to nervous and hormonal influences. In the opossum the basal tone occurs independently of extrinsic nervous activity as indicated by the lack of effect of extrinsic denervation. *In vitro*, tone in the lower oesophageal sphincter continues after treatment with tetrodotoxin to block nervous conduction excluding also the intrinsic nerves as the source of basal tone. The situation is quite different in both dog and cat since vagotomy has been reported to have dramatic effects ranging from decrease in resting tone to increase or muscular spasm. This variability is due to the existence of both excitatory and inhibitory pathways in the vagus nerves to this region. In the cat, excitatory responses to vagal stimulation are blocked by atropine and hexamethonium illustrating a classical parasympathetic innervation. After atropine, however, electrical stimulation of the vagus nerves results in relaxation of the circular muscle layer which is followed by a 'rebound' contraction after stimulation has stopped.

Atropine consistently reduced sphincter tone in the dog by 20–30%. Spontaneous discharge in the vagal cholinergic pathway therefore contributes to basal tone. However, one cannot quantify precisely the vagal cholinergic contribution for two reasons. Firstly, after atropine the balance between the excitatory and inhibitory pathways is lost so that the inhibitory pathways act unopposed. Secondly, sympathetic effects on the lower oesophageal sphincter are also modified by atropinization.

Stimulation of the sympathetic innervation to the lower oesophageal sphincter in the cat does not cause relaxation, as it does in the stomach, but contracts the sphincter (Gonella, Neil and Roman, 1979). This effect is mediated through alpha-adrenoreceptors and is blocked by phentolamine or depletion of transmitter stores in the noradrenergic nerve terminals by treatment with 6-hydroxydopamine. Both treatments can cause up to a 20% reduction in basal tone. Beta-adrenoreceptors have also been demonstrated, but when activated these inhibit resting tone.

The observation that atropine greatly reduced the response to sympathetic stimulation was a surprising finding. It suggested that the sympathetic innervation may act in part by releasing acetylcholine from cholinergic myenteric nerves (see p. 69). This point was confirmed in experiments where the release of acetylcholine was estimated by measuring the output of radiolabelled acetylcholine from segments of lower oesophageal sphincter preincubated with tritiated choline (Figure 5.5). Noradrenaline stimulated this output via a synaptic action since the effect was abolished by treatments which restricted the availability of Ca^{2+} necessary for transmitter release. Since the release of acetylcholine was unaffected by the presence of tetrodotoxin in the bathing medium the noradrenaline would appear to act presynaptically on the cholinergic nerve terminals.

While neurogenic mechanisms are, therefore, implicated in the generation of resting tone in the dog and cat, hormones, especially gastrin, may play a role in generating tone in other species including man. Initial observations implicating gastrin stemmed from observations on the effect of injections of exogenous pentagastrin or gastrin-17 on lower oesophageal sphincter tone. However, these effects appear to be from pharmacological rather than physiological doses since only weak sphincteric contractions occur at doses giving maximum secretions of gastric acid. A more physiological role in man is associated with changes in tone during acidification or alkalination of the gastric mucosa, procedures which modify the release of endogenous gastrin. These findings, however, are countered by the observation of normal sphincter profiles in patients with Zollinger–Ellison syndrome who have a gastrin-secreting tumour. A physiological role for gastrin in determining sphincter pressure is indicated from the use of gastrin antisera which bind gastrin in the bloodstream and prevent it reaching its target receptors. In the opossum, lower oesophageal sphincter tone is markedly reduced by antigastrin treatment (see Goyal and Cobb, 1981).

Most other gastrointestinal hormones have also been tested on the lower oesophageal sphincter but as yet are not directly implicated in its regulation (Table 5.1). However, the interaction of some of these hormones on muscle tone and/or transmitter release may be responsible for the increased sphincter pressure seen following the ingestion of meals of different composition. The female reproductive hormones also have action on the lower oesophageal sphincter and are probably responsible for the pregnant woman's predisposition towards oesophageal reflux.

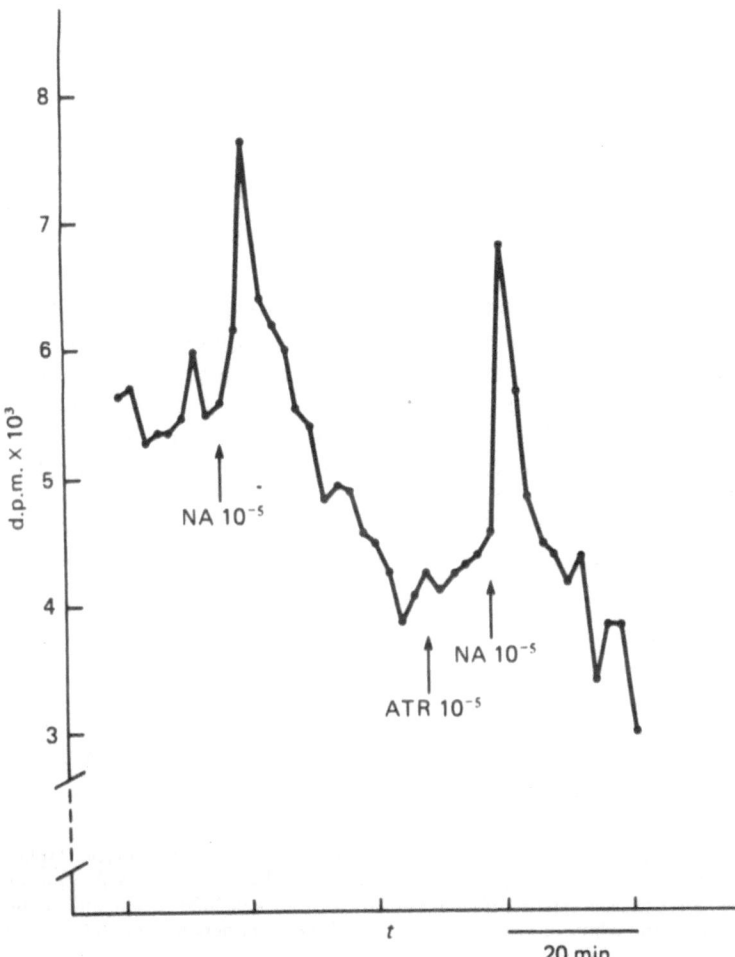

Figure 5.5 Output of radioactivity from lower oesophageal sphincter muscle strips loaded with tritiated choline. Noradrenaline (10^{-5}gml^{-1}) applied at arrows induced peaks in radioactivity indicating an increased release of acetylcholine. Atropine did not alter the output, the peaks were not, therefore, the result of mechanical expulsion of labelled molecules during noradrenaline induced contractions (From Gonella, Niel and Roman, 1980, with kind permission of the authors and the editor of J. Physiol. (London))

Sphincter relaxation

Relaxation of the lower oesophageal sphincter occurs during swallowing, oesophageal distension and vomiting as a consequence of activation of the vagal inhibitory innervation with release of its non-adrenergic, non-cholinergic transmitter (see Chapter 4). This contrasts with the upper oesophageal sphincter which relaxes when activity in its tonic motor innervation is temporarily interrupted. However, in the dog, which has a choli-

Table 5.1 Effect of gastrointestinal hormones on lower oesophageal sphincter tone

Hormones causing contraction	Hormones causing relaxation
Gastrin	Secretin
CCK	Glucagon
Motilin	VIP
SubstanceP	GIP
Pancreatic polypeptide	Somatostatin

nergic component to the basal spincter tone, Miolan and Roman (1978a) have suggested that relaxation also depends on inhibition of the excitatory cholinergic pathway. This hypothesis is based on the discharge characteristics of vagal efferent fibres recorded in conscious dogs by the reinnervated diaphragm technique (see p. 50). Two groups of neurones were identified whose firing was temporally correlated with lower oesophageal sphincter

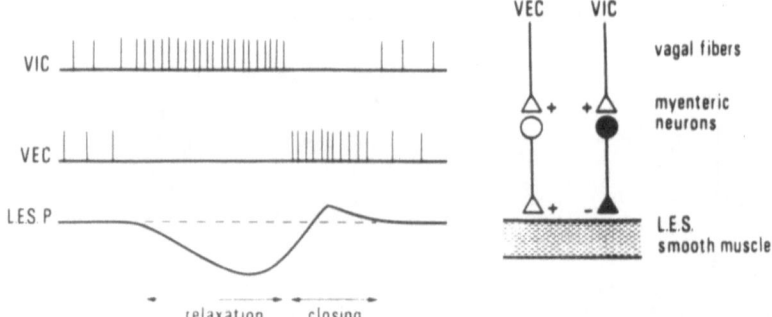

Figure 5.6 Schematic representation of the vagal control of the lower oesophageal sphincter. Symbols: VEC = vagal excitatory fibre; VIC = vagal inhibitory fibre; LES.P = pressure in the lower (o)esophageal sphincter (From Miolan and Roman, 1978a[139], with kind permission of the authors, the editor of J. Physiol. (Paris) and the publishers Masson S.A., Paris)

relaxation (Figure 5.6). The reciprocal relationship of the discharge in these two groups of neurones suggested that the two vagal pathways (excitatory and inhibitory) were reciprocally controlled. Increases in lower oesophageal sphincter pressure by procedures which interfered with the patency of the sphincter, for example the attempted withdrawal of a balloon against the closed sphincter, were also correlated with vagal discharge patterns which again were reciprocally modulated.

In species whose distal oesophagus is composed of smooth muscle, lower oesophageal sphincter relaxation can occur *in vitro*. The sphincter relaxation is associated with activation of the intramural inhibitory nerves as a consequence of the descending wave of inhibition which precedes the peristaltic contraction. Relaxation can therefore occur via activation of the intramural inhibitory nerves by both intrinsic and extrinsic reflexes (Figure 5.7).

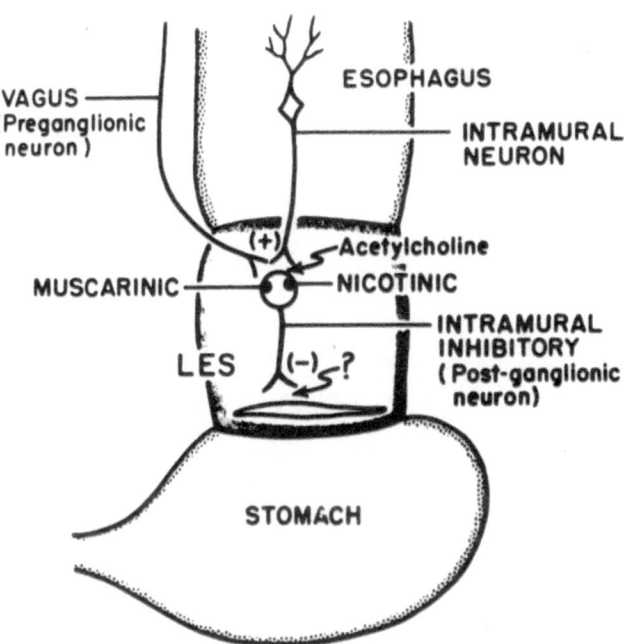

Figure 5.7 Diagrammatic representation of the major inhibitory pathways to the lower (o)esophageal sphincter (LES) (From Goyal and Cobb, 1981, with kind permission of the authors and publisher, Raven Press)

6
The stomach

INTRODUCTION

The diverse dietary adaptations that have evolved in different animals is represented in the range in complexity of their stomachs. Herbivores ingest plant fibre almost continuously, and this must be hydrolysed by bacteria to release the nutrients essential for life. In ruminants such as cow and

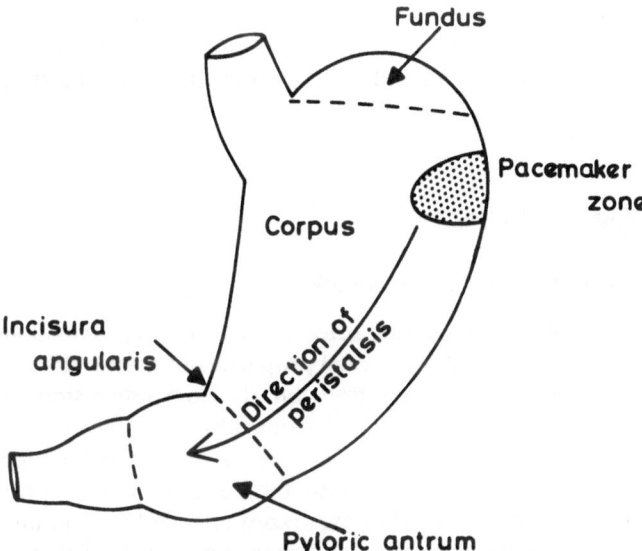

Figure 6.1 Stomach drawn diagrammatically to illustrate terminology used in text (From Grundy and Scratcherd, 1984, with kind permission of the publisher, Praeger)

sheep, this process takes place in the stomach (as opposed to the colons of other herbivores, see p. 127) which is considerably enlarged and compartmentalized. The forestomach, consisting of the reticulorumen is a fermentation drum which stores vast quantities (up to 200 litres in the cow) of pulped grass, swallowed saliva and symbiotic microorganisms. The products of this fermentation are absorbed through the epithelial lining of the foresto-mach and provide about 75% of the animal's daily energy requirement. From birth to when rumination develops, suckled milk is digested in the abomasum. This compartment additionally serves as a muscular pump which delivers digested milk in the preruminant animal or partially digested plant fibre in the weaned animal into the intestine.

In monogastric animals, including man, the bulk of digestion and absorp-tion takes place in the small intestine and so the stomach is a relatively simple organ. Its function is to break down solid food into small particles which are dispersed in liquid and delivered slowly into the duodenum. Although the stomach consists solely of a single compartment it can be separated into two regions which perform different mechanical functions. The first is the proximal part, the corpus and fundic regions (Figure 6.1), which act as a receptacle for food so that large meals can be taken relatively infrequently. To fulfil this role, the region is specially adapted to accommodating large volumes of food with only small increases in intragastric pressure, a process referred to as receptive relaxation. The second function of the stomach is performed by the distal corpus and antrum which serve as a muscular pump to break up food, mix it with gastric secretions and drive the semisolid chyme, in a controlled way, through the pyloric sphincter into the duodenum. In this chapter the control of these different but mutually related functions in the simple stomach are discussed.

THE PROXIMAL STOMACH

Properties of gastric smooth muscle

A cellular basis for the functional differences between proximal and distal stomach has been identified. Electrical properties of gastric smooth muscle have been studied by recording intracellularly from single smooth muscle cells that are part of a strip removed from different regions of stomach. This type of study has revealed a gradation of the resting membrane potential from fundus to antrum with the former being approximately 20 mV less negative than the latter (Szurszewski, 1981a). The importance of this observation becomes apparent when the relationship between resting membrane potential and tension generated by smooth muscle cells is considered (Figure 6.2). The fundic smooth muscle cells at their resting membrane potential are partially contracted. Thus, hyperpolarization of these cells will allow the muscle to relax and thereby increase the volume of this region. This is not the case in the antrum where the muscle is fully relaxed at the resting membrane potential and therefore will not relax

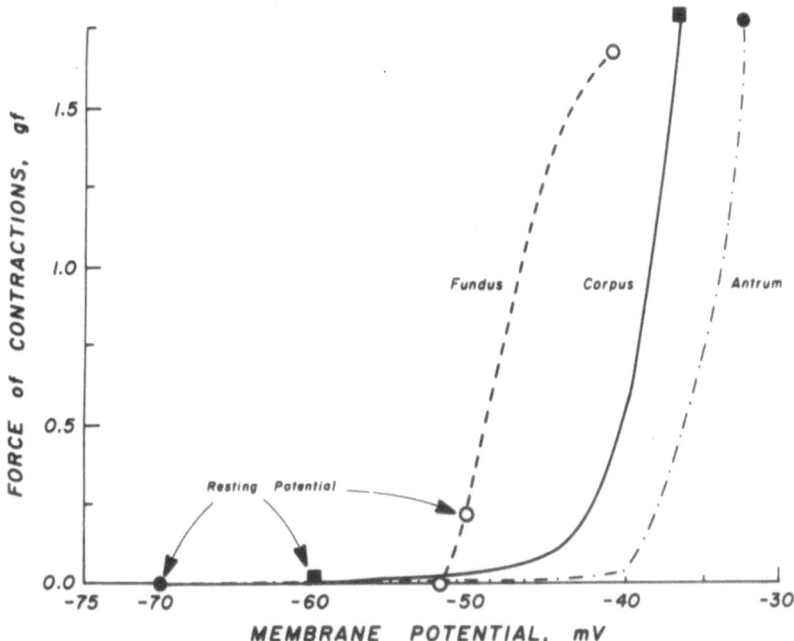

Figure 6.2 Comparison of voltage–tension curves of circular muscle from canine fundus, corpus and antrum. The measured values for resting membrane potential are also shown. Resting membrane potential in the fundus muscle is less negative than its threshold for contraction and so will develop spontaneous tone (From Szurszewski, 1981a, with kind permission of the author and publisher, Raven Press)

further when hyperpolarized. Thus the corpus has a capacity for relaxation which is absent in the antrum. Additionally, extrinsically denervated strips of muscle from these two regions, when subjected to stretch, show a different length–tension relationship so that the corpus generates much less tension when stretched than does the antrum (Figure 6.3). Thus, under isotonic conditions the muscle wall of the corpus will lengthen to a greater degree than the antrum. These two observations account for the distinction between antrum and corpus with regard to the stomach's reservoir function, so that over 80% of gastric contents are located in the corpus and fundus.

The reflex regulation of the proximal stomach

Parasympathetic reflexes

The inherent properties of smooth muscle in the proximal stomach are facilitated by reflexes which trigger receptive relaxation. The relaxation of the lower oesophageal sphincter that occurs during swallowing extends in to the stomach so that the pressure in the stomach falls as food is ingested. The timing of the relaxation is such that the lowest pressure occurs at

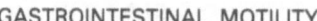

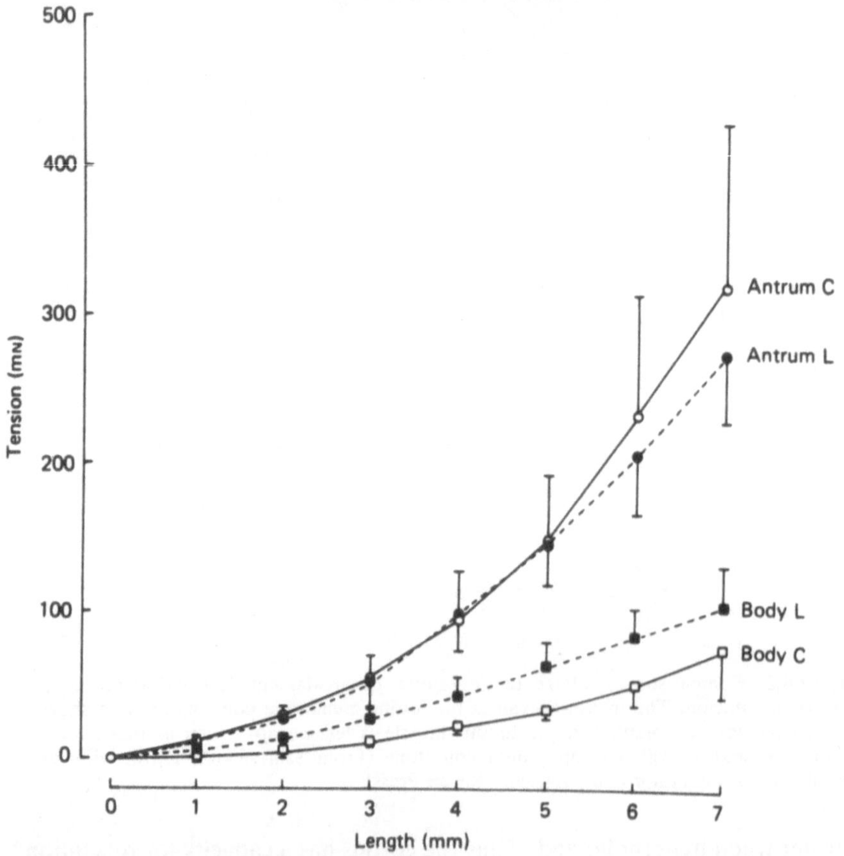

Figure 6.3 The length–tension relationship of strips of antral and corpus (body) regions of the stomach wall. C strips cut parallel to the circular axis, L strips cut parallel with the longitudinal axis (From Andrews *et al.*, 1980b, with kind permission of the the editor of J. Physiol. (London))

approximately the time the bolus enters the stomach, although with repeated swallows the pressure remains low throughout (Figure 6.4). The delivery of a bolus into the stomach is not a prerequisite for receptive relaxation since it occurs during sham feeding, when the bolus is diverted to the outside through an oesophagostomy, and oesophageal distension with a balloon. The afferent limb of the reflex is therefore activated from mechanoreceptors in the oesophagus which in turn enhance the discharge in the vagal inhibitory nerves to the stomach. Receptive relaxation can also be triggered by distension of the stomach itself (Abrahamsson and Jansson, 1973). Here, distension is again detected by the in-series tension receptors which also activates the vagal inhibitory pathway so that the pressure rise in the stomach is limited.

The various factors contributing to gastric accommodation have been

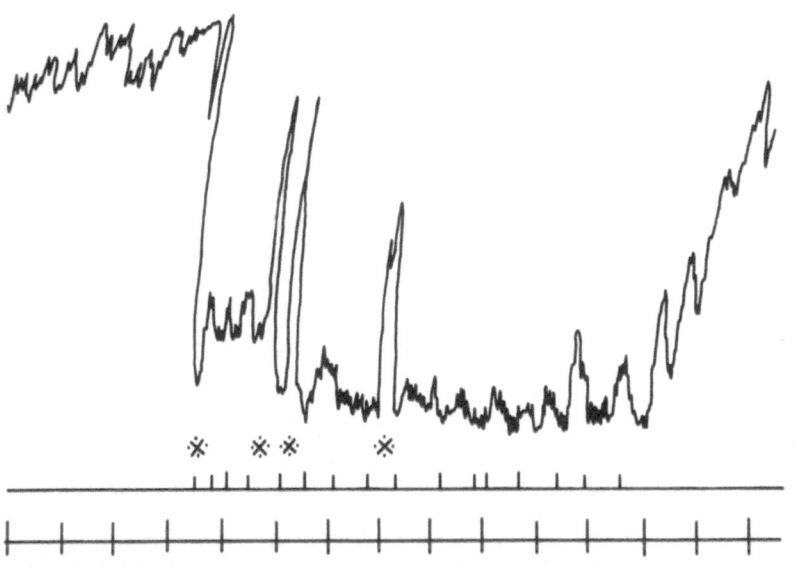

Figure 6.4 Continued gastric relaxation with repeated swallows. The upper trace shows gastric volume with a downward deflection indicating relaxation. The middle trace marks the act of swallowing; the bottom line, time in half-minutes. The asterisks indicate when the animal moved excitedly, causing rapid changes in gastric volume (From Cannon and Lieb, 1911, with kind permission of the editor of Am. J. Physiol.)

investigated by quantifying the intragastric pressure rise associated with the infusion of a fixed volume of fluid at a rate chosen to represent a physiological stimulus (Figure 6.5). The pressure in the stomach rises during the infusion and adapts slowly over the 2 min following the end of the infusion. After bilateral vagotomy the peak and adapted pressures are higher than controls but much lower after treatment with atropine. Activity in the vagus nerve, therefore, exerts a suppressive effect on the stomach helping to keep intragastric pressure low. However, since atropine reduces pressure there must also be cholinergic tone to the proximal stomach. Thus, it is possible that activation of vagally mediated relaxation via the inhibitory pathway may also involve the simultaneous suppression of activity in the antagonistic cholinergic pathway. The electrophysiological correlate of this has been described in the experiments in conscious dogs surgically prepared with a hemidiaphragm reinnervated with preganglionic vagal fibres (Miolan and Roman, 1974). Two distinct patterns of vagal activity were identified which correlated temporally with relaxation of the lower oesophageal sphincter and stomach elicited by swallowing or oesophageal distension. During receptive relaxation one vagal discharge pattern showed excitation while the other was being inhibited suggesting reciprocal control of the vagal excitatory and inhibitory pathways.

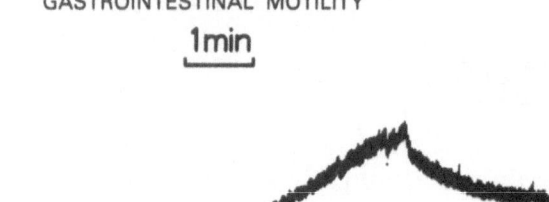

Figure 6.5 Intragastric pressure rises associated with slow $(10\,\text{ml}\,\text{min}^{-1})$ infusions of 50 ml of 0.9% NaCl solution. The lower trace is the control infusion with the volume being accommodated with only a small rise in intragastric pressure. After vagotomy (middle trace) a higher intragastric pressure results from the same volume distension. Section of the greater splanchnic nerves, after vagotomy, results in a further elevation in pressure during distension. Splanchnic section prior to vagotomy does not result in this increased pressure rise (Courtesy of Andrews, Grundy and Lawes)

The effectiveness of vagal reflexes in gastric accommodation can be gauged from the observation that intragastric pressure rarely exceeds 10 mmHg even during the ingestion of a large meal, although after ingestion the pressure in the corpus rises phasically to press gastric contents towards the antral pump (see Kelly, 1981). The solid component of a meal forms a mass in the proximal stomach which expands as more and more food is ingested. Because contractile activity in the proximal stomach is limited to tonal changes there is minimal mixing of contents so that seperate courses of a multicourse meals form distinct layers in the stomach lumen. Liquids, however, flow around the outside of the mass, rapidly enter the distal stomach and are then emptied into the duodenum. Hence, solid and liquid components of a meal empty at different rates.

Gastric relaxation also occurs during vomiting when the vagal inhibitory pathway is activated to allow the contracting abdominal muscles to expel gastric contents from a flaccid stomach (Abrahamsson, Jansson and Martinson, 1973). The vagal inhibitory pathway is also postulated to be involved, together with sympathetic reflexes, in the suppression of gastric motility seen following abdominal surgery (Abrahamsson, Glise and Glise, 1979). This condition is called 'paralytic ileus'.

Sympathetic reflexes

Discharge in the sympathetic fibres to the stomach also contribute to maintaining low intragastric pressures. Spinal reflexes activated by antral

(Abrahamsson, 1974) and intestinal (Jannson and Martinson, 1966) distension reduce gastric tone, although whether these stimuli occur naturally is not proven. There is an increase in gastric tone in conscious dogs following injection of guanethidine which blocks the release of noradrenaline from sympathetic nerve terminals (Jahnberg *et al.*, 1977) suggesting that spontaneous sympathetic activity is normally present and that removing this causes an increase in tone. A similar conclusion was reached by Andrews, Grundy and Lawes (1980), but in this study a significant increase in pressure following section of the greater splanchnic nerve was only seen after prior section of the vagus or prior treatment with atropine (see Figure 6.5). The action of tonic activity in the sympathetic nerves on intragastric pressure would appear, therefore, to be suppressed by the vagal cholinergic pathway in a way indicative of presynaptic modulation (see p. 69).

THE DISTAL STOMACH

Properties of gastric smooth muscle

Just as the proximal stomach is adapted to act as a reservoir for storing food, the distal stomach has properties suited to its function as a mechanical pump. Thus the distal, but not proximal stomach shows myogenic oscillations in resting membrane potential that forms the basis for antral contractions. In isolated segments of gastric muscle the intrinsic slow wave frequency shows a gradient from proximal to distal regions with the highest frequency being generated at a point on the greater curve in the midcorpus region (see Figure 6.1) This region, therefore, acts as a pacemaker for more distal regions so that in the intact stomach only one frequency is seen. The extracellular correlate of these intracellular potentials can be detected from electrodes implanted on the serosal surface of the stomach. These record electrical potentials which appear to propagate through the antrum at a velocity which increases as it approaches the pylorus (Figure 6.6). The slow waves or pacesetter potentials have a characteristic waveform. When recorded with intracellular electrodes they resemble the cardiac action potential with a rapid depolarization and maintained plateau potential (Figure 6.7). Extracellularly, a brief triphasic complex is followed by a much longer isoelectric potential with the whole cycle recurring at the slow wave frequency. The amplitude of individual contractions is determined by the amplitude and duration of the plateau potentials which are themselves dependent upon external nervous and hormonal influences (Figure 6.8). In more distal antral regions the plateau potentials commonly have spike activity, which contributes towards the generation of a contraction, superimposed on the plateau potential (see Figure 6.7). These are also detected extracellularly as spike bursts during the isoelectric phase, and are frequently used as an index of contractile activity (Figure 6.9).

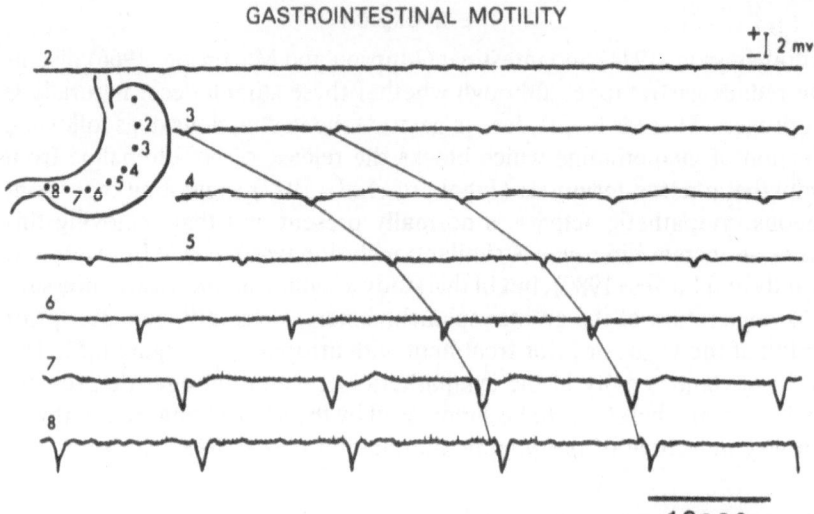

Figure 6.6 Electrical activity recorded from electrodes on the surface of the stomach (position shown in inset). Slow waves or pacesetter potentials occur continuously at about 12s intervals and appear to spread caudally from the mid-corpus region with increasing velocity (From Kelly, Code and Elveback, 1969, with kind permission of the authors and the editor of Am. J. Physiol.)

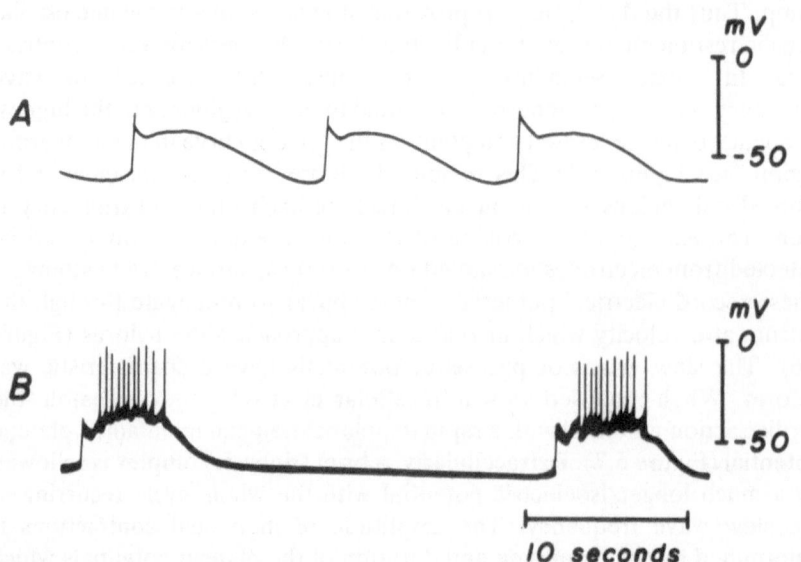

Figure 6.7 Intracellular electrical activity recorded from circular muscle of human stomach. A:Orad atrum. B: Terminal antrum (From Szurszewski, 1981, with kind permission of the author and publisher, Raven Press)

Patterns of antral contractility

Antral contractions originate in the mid-corpus region and propagate

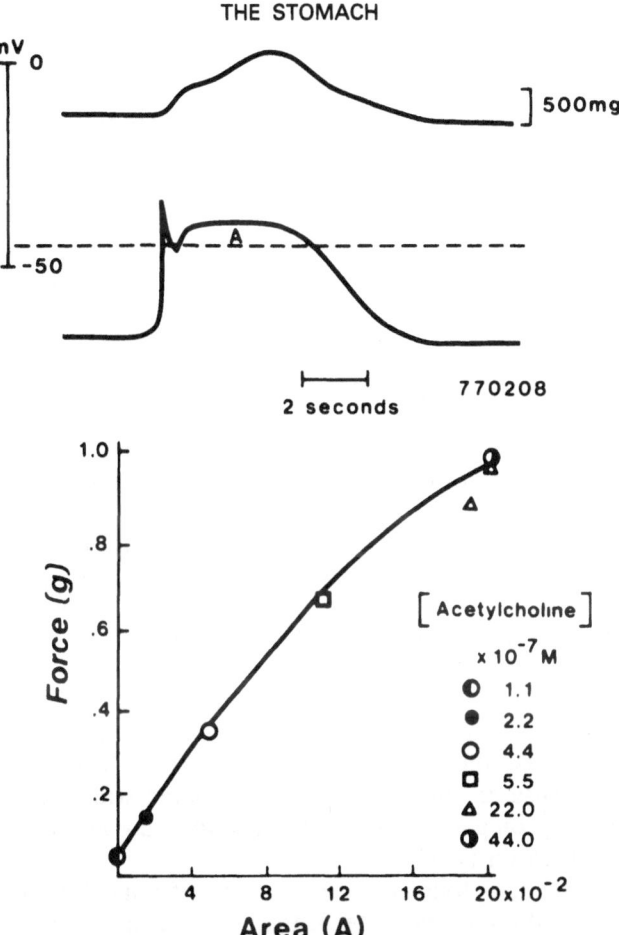

THE STOMACH

770208

2 seconds

Figure 6.8 - Relationship between voltage–time interval (area A) and amplitude of contraction. Each point was obtained when steady-state response were achieved in the indicated concentration of acetylcholine (ACh). Top trace, contraction; bottom trace, intracellularly recorded action potential. Dashed line represents the voltage threshold for contraction (From Szurszewski, 1981, with kind permission of the author and publisher, Raven Press)

caudally towards the pylorus as a ring of contraction. The frequency of contractions is determined by the omnipresent slow waves while the amplitude depends on extrinsic influences modifying the amplitude of the plateau potentials (Szurszewski, 1977b). In man gastric contractions occur at about $3\,min^{-1}$ while in the dog the frequency is $5\,min^{-1}$. The force generated by individual antral contractions varies enormously. When measured with a catheter in the gastric lumen the amplitude of phasic pressure waves varies from barely detectable to over $100\,mmHg$ with the latter representing a powerful propulsive force. The full range of antral activity can be seen in the fasted animal which shows the cyclical motor pattern

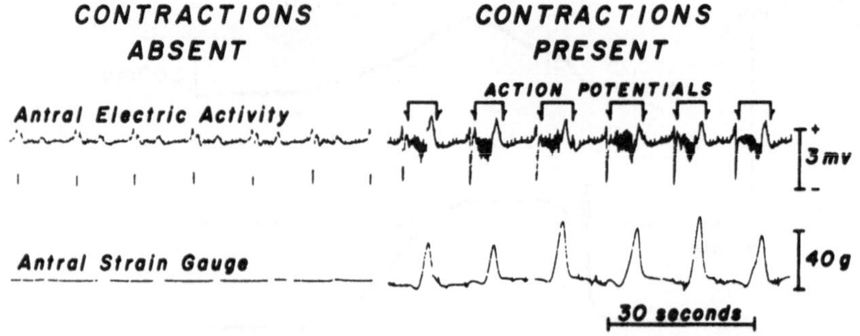

Figure 6.9 Relationship between extracellularly recorded electrical activity and antral contractions (From Kelly, 1976, with kind permission of the author and the editor of Viewpoints on Dig. Dis.)

associated with the migration of a motor complex from stomach to terminal ileum (see Chapter 9). Antral contractions are absent for 1–2 hours after which contractions appear and build up to a short period of intense peristaltic activity lasting 20–30 min before the stomach again returns to quiescence. The intense phase is referred to as the activity front or phase III and is responsible for the complete evacuation of any gastric contents that may have built up during the quiescent phase; even large particles which are not emptied during the postprandial phase are emptied during these activity fronts. They are, therefore, suggested to have a 'housekeeper' function which periodically sweeps the bowel clean (Code and Schlegel, 1974). The intense gastric contractions associated with phase III of the migrating motor complex probably correspond to the hunger contractions described by Carlson (1916).

Antral contractions following the ingestion of a meal do not show the cyclical pattern of the fasted state. If the antrum is quiescent then feeding stimulates contractions of only moderate amplitude although the level of motility is extremely variable and depends upon the volume and composition of the meal. These contractions are the driving force for the emptying of the meal into the duodenum, and together with contractions of the pylorus and duodenum determine the rate at which gastric contents are emptied into the duodenum. The contractile activity in the duodenum, pylorus and stomach are subjected to feedback mechanisms from the small intestine which adjust gastric emptying so that the digestive and absorptive capacity of the intestine is not overloaded. The mechanisms responsible for the conversion from fasted to fed motor activity are discussed in Chapter 10.

The reflex control of antral motility

Antral motility is reflexly stimulated by distension of the stomach. The reflex is triggered by stretch of the in-series tension receptors mainly in the corpus and fundic regions and activate the vagal cholinergic pathway to the antrum. This corpoantral reflex occurs when the stomach is completely

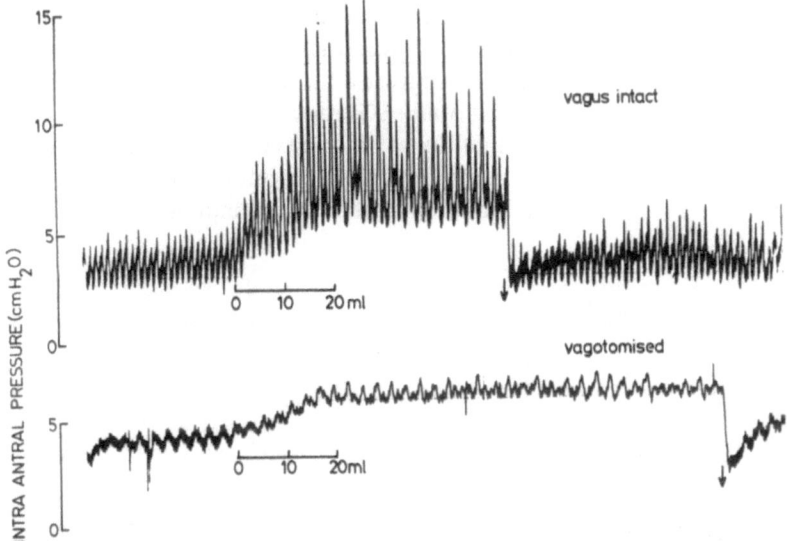

Figure 6.10 Above: the effect of inflation of the corpus region of a divided stomach on the pressure recorded from the antral compartment in an anaesthetized ferret. Note that as the volume in the corpus increased, large waves of contraction were evoked in the antrum. On deflation of the corpus (↓) the antral contractions immediately returned to a basal level. After bilateral cervical vagotomy (lower trace) there was no stimulation of antral motility by corpus inflation. The gradual increase in intra-antral pressure during corpus inflation is due to mechanical interference by the distended corpus (From Andrews, Grundy and Scratcherd,1980a, with kind permission of the the editor of J. Physiol. (London))

divided across the incisura and is abolished by vagotomy (Figure 6.10). The increase in antral contractions is proportional to the degree of corpus distension, and as the former is the driving force for gastric emptying it seems likely that this reflex accounts for the rate of gastric emptying being proportional to the volume of the meal (Hunt and Macdonald, 1954). There is, however, a time-lag following ingestion of a meal and the start of gastric emptying. A possible explanation for this is that during ingestion, receptive relaxation will temporarily reduce the afferent traffic from the corpus so that the reflex is only activated as the tone increases while the inhibitory influence is wearing off. Also, as the tone in the proximal stomach increases gastric contents are forced towards the distal pump and this facilitates emptying.

Inhibition of antral motility can be elicited by distension of any region of small or large intestine, a reflex mediated via the splanchnic nerves and abolished by adrenoreceptor blockade. Such a reflex switches off all gastrointestinal motility and is probably a protective mechanism activated by intestinal obstruction. The discharge of vagal efferent fibres is also inhibited by intestinal distension, a reflex whose afferent input is via a non-vagal pathway suggesting a possible splanchnovagal contribution to the suppression of gut motility under pathological conditions. However, only low threshold volumes were necessary to elicit the reflex inhibition of vagal efferent discharge (with pressures lower than those occurring naturally during contractions), which may suggest a more physiological role in the feedback regulation of antral motility (Grundy and Scratcherd, 1982).

Reflex inhibition of antral motility can also be elicited by the stimulation of chemoreceptors in the small intestine. The infusion of acid into the duodenum has a powerful inhibitory effect on antral motility while simulta-

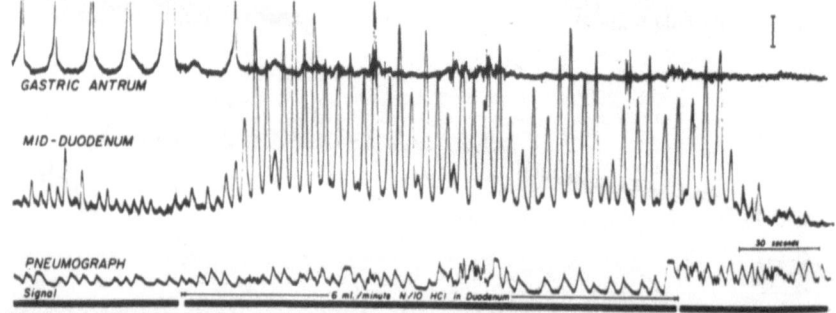

Figure 6.11 Effect of duodenal instillation of acid (HCl 100 mmol/l at 6 ml min⁻¹) on gastric and duodenal motor activity in the fasting dog. Bar = 25 cmH₂O (From Brink, Schlegal and Code, 1965, with kind permission of the authors and the editor of Gut)

neously enhancing duodenal contractions (Figure 6.11). The short latency of the response and its dependence on an intact vagus point towards a neural reflex. Indeed the discharge of vagal efferent fibres is markedly reduced when acid is instilled into the duodenum (see Roman and Gonella, 1981). The physiological importance of this reflex is uncertain since continuous measurements of duodenal pH indicate that the pH rarely falls low enough to stimulate such a reflex, and when it does it is only transient because of the release of secretin which increases the output of pancreatic bicarbonate to buffer the acid. However, since testmeals with an acidic pH empty more slowly from the stomach than neutral meals it would seem reasonable to conclude that such a reflex serves to prevent the buffering capacity of the duodenum from being overloaded. Yet treatment with histamine H_2-receptor antagonists, which inhibit endogenous acid production, does not affect the rate of gastric emptying suggesting that the quantity of endogenous acid delivered to the duodenum is not an important regulator of gastric emptying (Heading *et al.*, 1977).

The pyloric sphincter

The pyloric sphincter is a physically recognizable structure consisting of two loops of muscle of which the distal loop is the most prominent (Figure

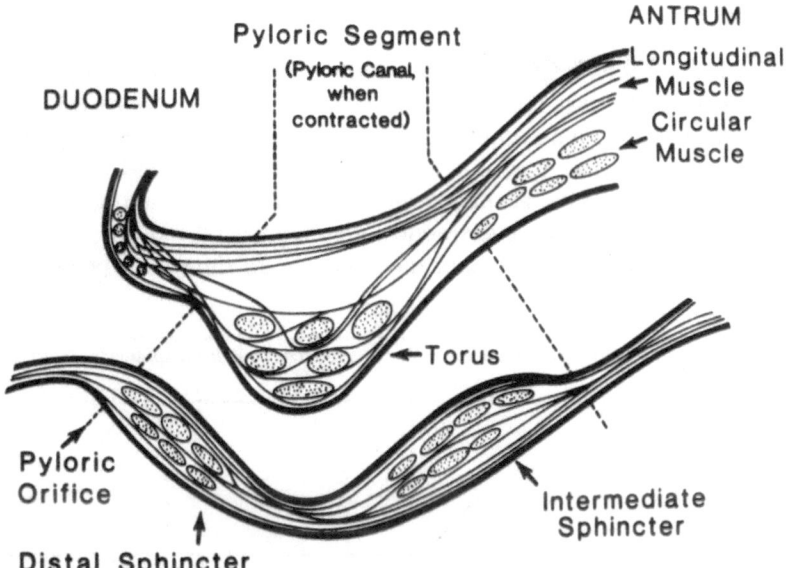

Figure 6.12   Longitudinal section through the gastroduodenal junction giving a scheme of its muscular anatomy (From Schulze-Delrieu, Wright and Shirazi, 1984, with kind permission of the authors and publisher, MTP Press)

6.12). It plays an important role in the controlled delivery of chyme (liquefied food mixed with gastric secretions) into the duodenum and also helps limit the reflux of bile into the stomach. It differs from the lower oesophageal sphincter, which is usually kept closed, because it opens and closes in phase with antral contractions. The pylorus is open as the wave of contraction propagates through the proximal antrum but as the contraction approaches the terminal antrum it closes so that emptying ceases and the antral contents are forced backwards into the proximal antrum. Thus the pylorus is closed when the peristaltic wave reaches it; this traps gastric contents between the wave of contraction and the pylorus and allows only liquids and small particles to escape through the narrow pyloric canal. Larger particles are retropelled facilitating both their mechanical breakdown and dispersion in liquid.

The luminal diameter of the pyloric canal can be modified independently of the antral waves. This region is richly innervated from both parasympathetic and sympathetic divisions of the autonomic nervous system. As is the case in the lower oesophageal sphincter, alpha-adrenoreceptor activation constrict the sphincter and contribute to the baseline tone of the muscle which in turn determines the pyloric diameter during the open phase of the antral contractions. VIP-like immunoreactivity has been detected in the pylorus and may be responsible for nerve-mediated inhibition of sphincter tone (Edin, 1980).

HORMONAL REGULATION

The hormonal influences on gastric motility are poorly understood. The plasma levels of several of the gastrointestinal hormones increase following the ingestion of food, and while many of these have primary effects on other systems – for example gastric and pancreatic secretion, and gallbladder contractions – they have also been implicated in the normal regulation of gastric motility. The major hormones affecting gastric motility and their effects on the different regions of the stomach are shown in Table 6.1.

Table 6.1 Effect of hormones on gastric motility

	Proximal stomach	Distal stomach	Pyloric sphincter	Gastric emptying
Gastrin	–	+	+	–
CCK	–	+	+	–
Secretin	–	–	+	–
Glucagon	–	–	+	–
GIP	–	–	+	–

– = relaxation: + = contraction

The common feature of all these hormones is their inhibitory effects on gastric emptying, achieved by relaxing the proximal stomach and increasing tone in the pyloric sphincter. The effects on antral motility are more varied with gastrin and CCK both stimulating contractions. In addition, gastrin causes an approximately 20% increase in the slow wave frequency and speeds up antral contractions. The effects listed above are generally associated with infusions of exogenous hormone into the bloodstream, and in many cases the plasma levels required to elicit an effect exceed those normally encountered postprandially. From a physiological viewpoint, CCK is probably the most important hormone involved in the feedback regulation of gastric emptying since inhibition of emptying occurs at similar doses required for gallbladder and pancreatic responses. The hormone motilin is considered in Chapter 9 in relation to the control of the migrating motor complex.

GASTRIC EMPTYING

The actual process of gastric emptying, especially of solid meals, involves a coordinated sequence of contractions of antrum, pyloric sphincter and duodenum. The proximal stomach acts as a 'hopper' to deliver food into the antral pump so that solids are broken down to fine particles which are dispersed in liquid before being emptied into the duodenum. Liquid and solid components of a meal are emptied at different rates even when ingested simultaneously and are said to depend on different control mechanisms such that the emptying of solids is a function of the antrum, while the emptying of liquids depends upon the pressure gradient between proximal stomach and duodenum. This distinction is based on the observation that truncal vagotomy inhibits the emptying of solids while promoting the emptying of liquids (Cooke, 1975). Vagotomy reduces the amplitude of the antral contractions by removing the excitatory cholinergic tone and thereby slows down the breakdown of solids and their subsequent emptying. By removing the vagal inhibitory nerves to the proximal stomach receptive relaxation is prevented and the consequent increase in pressure gradient between stomach and duodenum facilitates the emptying of liquids. Since the pyloric sphincter generally constricts as a part of the coordinated sequence of the antral wave, after vagotomy the sphincter remains open thereby allowing liquids to empty quickly.

The relationship between antral motility, pyloric opening and duodenal contractions has been studied in conscious animals by recording electrical events from serosal electrodes or mechanical events from strain gauges attached to the serosal surface. In addition the sequence of events can be monitored using cineradiographic techniques to visualize the emptying of contrast medium from the stomach. Using a combination of these techniques Ehrlein, Keinke and Schemann (1984) have differentiated three phases of gastric emptying with each antral wave (Figure 6.13). The propulsive phase occurs mainly as the peristaltic wave spreads over the mid-antral region. The terminal antrum is relaxed and the pyloric orifice is opening to its widest so that resistance to flow is low and gastric contents flow into the duodenum. As the the wave of contraction propagates towards the pyloric sphincter, gastric contents are either emptied through the open pylorus or retropelled into more proximal regions. In this phase, therefore, evacuation and retropulsion occur simultaneously. The less powerful the contractions, the wider is the antral lumen at the point of contraction, and consequently the more chyme is forced backwards as the wave approaches the terminal antrum. With the development of the terminal antral contraction, the pyloric sphincter closes and emptying no longer occurs. The powerful antral contractions grind the luminal contents which are forced back into the proximal antrum. The duodenum contracts two or three times during each antral wave and is coordinated, probably via the enteric plexuses, so that the just-emptied chyme is rapidly whisked along to the distal duodenum and jejunum. Uncoordinated duodenal contractions impair emptying by increasing the resistance to flow.

Lower viscosity meals empty more quickly than meals of higher viscosity because the amplitude of antral contractions and therefore the degree to which the contraction occlude the lumen is greater with the low viscosity meal (Prove and Ehrlein, 1982). With highly viscous stomach contents, the tension in the wall of the antrum during contraction will be greater. Excessive tension, as detected by antral mechanoreceptors, could reflexly

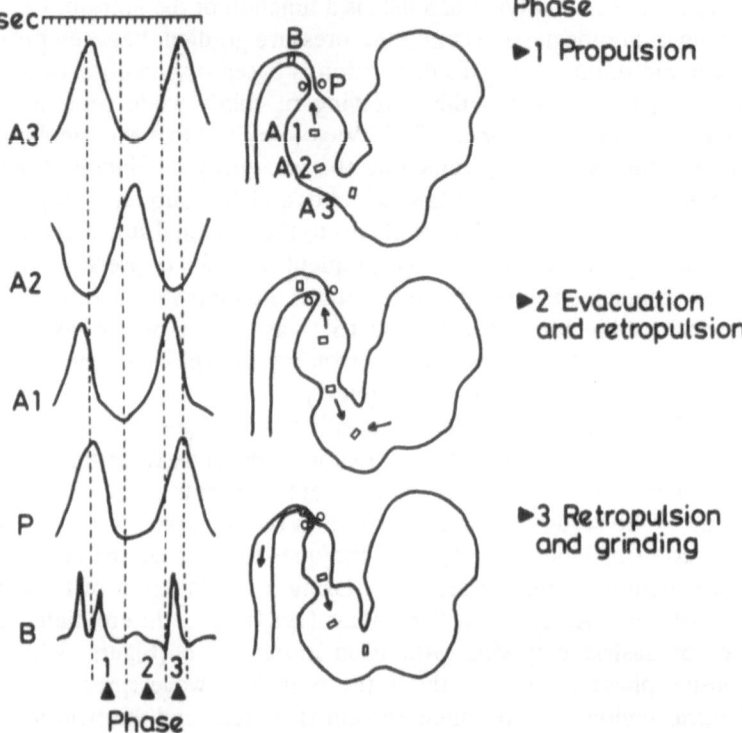

Figure 6.13 Relationship between gastroduodenal contractions and flow of digesta. The traces on the left relate to the strain gauges attached at the positions shown. A = antrum, P = pyloric sphincter, B = duodenal bulb. On the right are the outlines of the gastroduodenal region during propagated antral contractions and the phases of gastric emptying determined by cineradiography. See text for details (Modified from Ehrlein and Akkermans, 1984, with the authors' corrections)

limit the strength of individual contractions by a mechanism involving the vagal efferent innervation to this region (see p. 51). Some of these efferent fibres show a differential response to low and high threshold afferent stimulation such that an enhanced discharge is suppressed as the tension in the wall of the antrum increases further. If the discharge in these efferent fibres stimulated antral activity then its suppression at high tension would reduce the strength of antral contractions, and thereby the degree of antral indentation of gastric contents, and so reduce gastric emptying.

Tone in the proximal stomach facilitates emptying by gently squeezing gastric contents into the antral pump. Relaxation of the fundus and corpus will, therefore, result in gastric contents being retained in the proximal stomach and thereby reduce emptying.

Gastric emptying studies in man

The direct measurement of gastric volume following the ingestion of a test meal provides a simple method of quantifying the overall effect of the various factors contributing to gastric emptying. The techniques employed range in complexity. The simplest involve intubation procedures where samples of gastric contents are aspirated following the introduction of an inert marker such as phenol red so that the volume can be calculated from its dilution. Modern isotope techniques are less invasive and have the advantage of allowing the ingestion of normal meals as opposed to liquid test meals which obviously empty much more quickly; however, the latter do require the use of expensive gamma cameras and on-line computer analysis to evaluate the pattern of gastric emptying. The normal emptying profile is almost linear for solid meals while liquid emptying is more

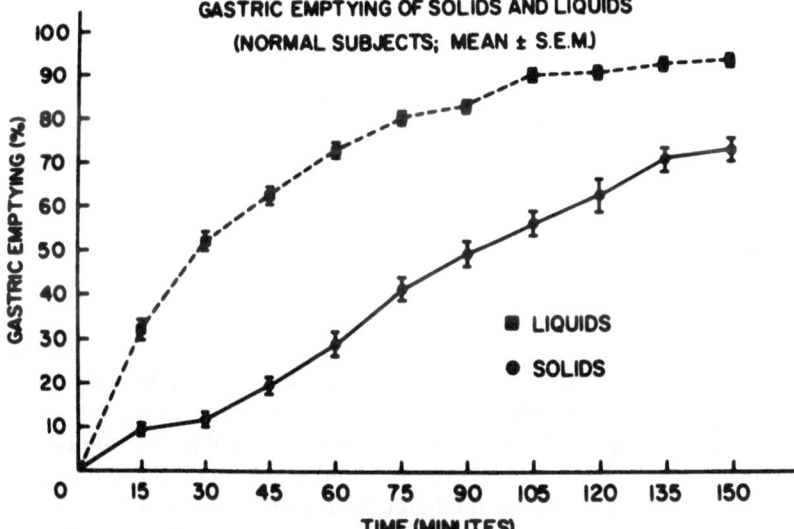

Figure 6.14 Gastric emptying curves of solid and liquid components of a mixed meal (From Malmud *et al.*, 1982, Scintigraphic evaluation of gastric emptying. *Seminars in Nuclear Medicine*, **XII**, 116–125, with kind permission from the authors and editor)

exponential (Figure 6.14). Large indigestible solids are not emptied during the postprandial period but are forced out of the stomach as the powerful phase III contractions develop in the interdigestive state.

Feedback regulation of gastric emptying

Receptors in the proximal small intestine detect the composition of the just-emptied chyme and generally act as a brake on the emptying process. Acidity, osmolarity and the concentration of nutrients in the chyme all reduce the rate of gastric emptying. The greater the concentration of acid in the chyme, the slower it is emptied from the stomach. Receptors have been identified which respond to acid, and from the rapidity of the response to acid in the duodenum one might suspect a neural mechanism. However, acid in the intestines causes the release of secretin which could also inhibit gastric emptying by the effects described above.

Osmoreceptors located in the duodenum and jejunum are postulated to shrink and swell depending on the osmolarity of luminal contents relative to intracellular osmolarity. As their volume changes they activate mechanisms which slow down the rate of gastric emptying. The receptors are thought to lie in the brush border of the intestinal villi since isocalorific meals of starch and glucose empty from the stomach at similar rates even though they are osmotically very different (Hunt and Knox, 1968). The starch must therefore be broken down to its composite monosaccharides before interacting with the osmoreceptors, and since the enzymes responsible for this final breakdown lie in the brush border it follows that the receptors must also be at this site. In patients with pancreatic insufficiency, starch empties more quickly since the pancreatic amylase necessary for the breakdown of polysaccharides to disaccharides is absent.

Proteins, like carbohydrates, are also emptied at a rate consistent with the products of hydrolysis acting on osmoreceptors. Osmoreceptors have been described with afferent fibres in the vagus nerves suggesting that their effect on gastric emptying is mediated through a neural mechanism. Certainly the delayed gastric emptying brought about by osmotic stimuli is abolished by vagotomy but since this procedure also disrupts antral contractility one cannot conclude that a vagal reflex is responsible.

Fats on the other hand exert their braking effect via receptors detecting the presence of fatty acids in the intestinal lumen. Triglyceride does not slow gastric emptying when administered to patients with pancreatic insufficiency or when bile is diverted from the duodenal lumen indicating that the breakdown product of fats is the stimulus. The inhibition of gastric emptying by fats may in part be mediated by the liberation of CCK, which at physiological levels causes relaxation of the proximal stomach and constriction of the pyloric sphincter. A hypothesis put forward by Hunt and Stubbs (1975) proposes that the calorific content of chyme determines the rate of gastric emptying; the higher the calorific density the greater the degree of slowing. Thus the receptors mediating feedback inhibition are proposed to be finely tuned so that the same degree of inhibition occurs irrespective of the source of calories.

Until recently, the receptors mediating feedback inhibition of gastric emptying were considered to be limited to the duodenum and jejunum. However, the introduction of fat emulsions into the distal ileum also delays gastric emptying, a phenomenon referred to as the 'ileal brake' (Read *et al.*, 1984). Thus receptors throughout the small intestine probably play an important role in regulating gastric emptying in such a way as to optimize intestinal digestion and absorption.

7
The small intestine

INTRODUCTION

The small intestine is the region of the digestive system where most of the enzymatic breakdown of food takes place and where the nutrients released from this breakdown are absorbed along with water and electrolytes. The mucosal and submucosal layers are particularly adapted to these digestive and absorptive functions; so too is the organization of small intestine motility. Contractions are of two main types. Segmentary contractions are the mixing movements which ensure dispersion of the various secretions from the liver, pancreas and intestinal surface throughout the chyme and also bring recently digested nutrients into contact with the absorptive surface. Peristaltic contractions propagate aborally for short distances and, together with the segmentary waves, keep digesta moving in an aboral direction.

In man the small intestine occupies about 75–80% of the total length of the digestive system and is divided into duodenum, jejunum and ileum. The duodenum is the first 25 cm of intestine, starting at the pylorus, and is morphologically distinct from the rest being devoid of mesentery and containing mucus-secreting Brunner's glands in the submucosal layer. The remaining 5 meters or so of small intestine is a coiled tube arbitrarily divided into jejunum (proximal two-fifths) and ileum (distal three-fifths). The chyme entering the duodenum from the stomach takes 2–4 hours to complete its journey to the terminal ileum with the exact transit time depending on both the volume and composition of the meal ingested. Although the motor function is basically the same throughout the small intestine the luminal contents become less bulky and more viscous as absorption continues. Associated with this change, but not necessarily as a consequence of it, are quantitative differences between proximal and distal regions with regard to frequency and patterns of contraction and a resultant decrease in the velocity of transit in more distal regions.

The myogenic properties of small intestinal smooth muscle and their

111

control by the intramural nerve plexuses together provide the basic mechanisms for segmentation and peristalsis (see Chapters 1 and 2). This chapter is limited to a discussion of the various patterns of small intestinal contractile activity and their control.

MOTOR PATTERNS AND THE FLOW OF DIGESTA

Interest in small intestinal motility over the past 15 years has concentrated on the phenomenon of the 'migrating motor complex' (MMC) and its disruption following the ingestion of food. Since these motor patterns are not limited only to the small intestine, but are a general feature of the proximal gastrointestinal tract, they are dealt with separately (see Chapters 9 and 10). However, with specific regard to the small intestine, the motility seen during the fasted and fed states illustrates the full spectrum of activity of the intestinal musculature.

In the fasted animal, motility at a single locus oscillates between two extremes, varying from complete inactivity through a period of irregular activity to a phase of intense contractile activity where each slow wave is

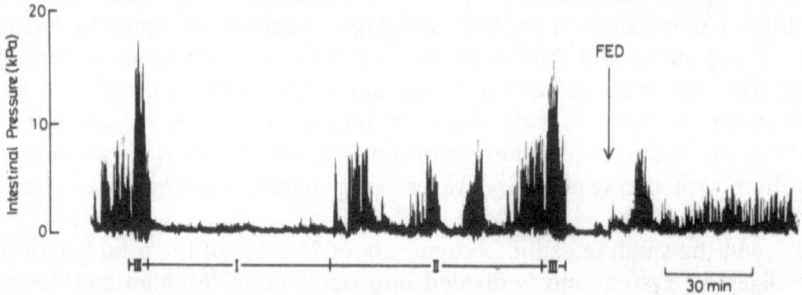

Figure 7.1 Jejunal motility recorded manometrically from a dog. Before the animal was fed (at arrow) a cyclical pattern of motility was evident while after feeding continuous contractile activity persisted for several hours. The numerals refer to phases of the migrating motor complex (MMC) (Courtesy of Bull, Grundy and Scratcherd)

associated with a contraction (Figure 7.1). The terminology used to describe fasting motor activity is taken from Code and Marlett's (1975) study in the conscious dog, but the description is also valid for man. Phase I is the inactive phase and continues for 30–60 min; phase II is the irregular phase and lasts for a similar length of time; intense contractile activity lasts for only 4–7 min and is referred to as phase III or the activity front. The whole cycle lasts for 80–120 min and is repeated indefinitely until feeding occurs. When several loci are viewed simultaneously this activity is seen to propagate along the the small intestine (Figure 7.2). The time taken for the complexes to propagate the length of the small intestine is approximately the same as the total cycle time so that contractile activity is always present

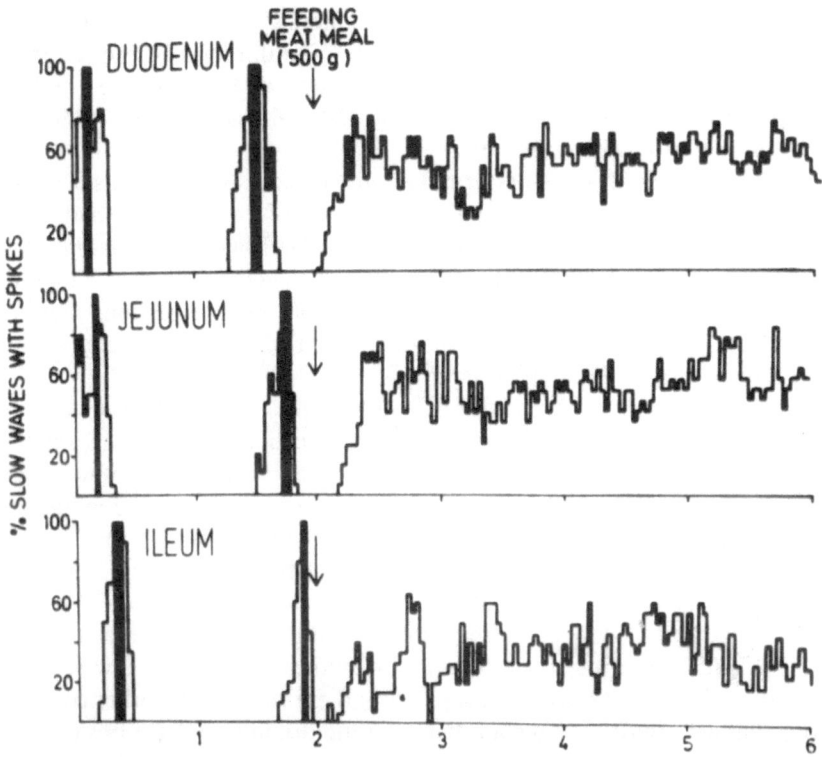

Figure 7.2 Fasting and fed motor activity recorded myoelectrically from three sites along the dog small intestine. Contractile activity is expressed as the % of slow waves with spikes: 0% = represents no contractions; 100% = spikes on every slow wave indicative of phase III of the MMC (black bar) (From Konturek, 1984, with kind permission of the author and publisher, MTP Press)

at some point in the small intestine (see also Figure 9.1, p. 147). The velocity at which the complex propagates is higher in more proximal regions travelling at 3.5–6.2 cm min⁻¹ in the jejunum and only 1.2–1.9 cm min⁻¹ in the terminal ileum. This means that the length of intestine simultaneously undergoing phase III activity becomes shorter in progressively distal regions. Similar MMC cycles are recorded from the small intestine of herbivores and therefore represent a basic motor pattern in all species. There are, however, species differences. In the sheep, for example, the velocity of propagation is very much higher but because the small bowel is also considerably longer the total cycle length is the same (Grivel and Ruckebusch, 1972). The other major difference is seen upon the ingestion of food. *Ad libitum* eaters, such as the cow and sheep, show continuous MMC activity. In animals that eat discrete meals, however, the ingestion of food is accompanied by the disappearance of the migrating motor complex. It is replaced by a continuous, irregular pattern of motility, similar in appearance to phase II activity, but present simultaneously along the whole length of small intestine (see Figure 7.1 and 7.2). The duration of the fed state depends upon the species studied, the volume of food ingested and its composition. In man a mixed meal of 450 kcal disrupts the MMC for 3.5 hours (Vantrappen *et al.*, 1977).

Before these contractile patterns were recognized as characteristic of the fasted and fed state, individual components of this activity had been described, but the authors questioned the variability of intestinal motility without realizing the cyclical nature of motor activity in the conscious animal. Consequently, early investigations on small intestinal motility concentrated on descriptions of the waveform of individual contractions and their effect on luminal contents.

At the beginning of this century Cannon (1902) used radiographic techniques on cats to examine the effects of intestinal contractions on the movement of contrast medium within the lumen. The most common type of motility observed under these conditions was rhythmic segmentation. This motor pattern is so described because contractions of the circular muscle layer appear to divide a loop of intestine into a series of short segments. Each narrow band of contraction has a frequency and duration determined by the slow wave frequency at that particular point (see below, p. 119) and forces intestinal contents in both directions. A few seconds later these initial contractions disappear and are replaced by other contractions that are almost equidistant between the original contractions (Figure

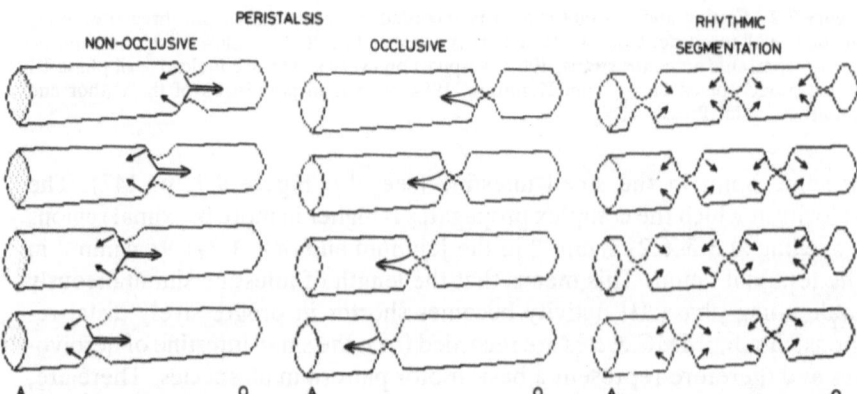

Figure 7.3 Computer simulation of peristalsis and segmentation. The sequence, from top to bottom, represents contractions in an intestinal segment frozen at equal intervals of time. The arrows indicate the movement of intestinal contents. A and O refer to the aboral and oral ends of the segment respectively

7.3). In this way short segments of intestine are repeatedly formed, divided and reformed. This type of motility is generally considered to be the mixing movements of the gut since at one point contents are forced in both directions. However, the aboral progression of these contractions has been documented. A length of intestine undergoing segmentation is seen to advance chyme aborally into regions of intestine that were previously quiescent.

In contrast to segmentary contractions, peristaltic waves are contractions which propagate along a length of bowel for a variable distance. If the force of contraction in the circular muscle layer is sufficient to occlude the intestinal lumen then propagation of the contraction caudally propels intestinal contents ahead of the wave (see Figure 7.3). Propulsion is aided in the respect by a descending wave of inhibition preceding the contraction (see Chapter 2). If contractions of the circular muscle are less powerful, so that the lumen is not occluded, then some of the intestinal contents will pass backwards through the narrow contracted region as the contraction propagates aborally and so aid mixing of luminal contents.

The effect of contractions of the longitudinal muscle layer on the flow of digesta are less easily visualized since they will move the intestinal wall in relation to the contents rather than the other way round. Contraction of the longitudinal muscle either proximally or distally to a band of contracted circular muscle will mix intestinal contents or force them in the direction of the contracting longitudinal muscle.

The proportion of the total contractile activity which was segmentary or peristaltic has been quantified in the jejunum of the conscious dog using spike activity recorded from closely spaced serosal electrodes as an index of contractile activity (Summers and Dusdieker, 1980). They distinguished segmental from peristaltic contractions by the temporal relationship of spike bursts at adjacent electrodes. Segmental contractions were associated with spike bursts that occurred at only one site, whereas during peristatic contractions the spike bursts propagated from one electrode to the next at a velocity determined by the aboral spread of slow wave activity (see p. 119). The proportion of either type of contractile activity varied with the fed and fasted state. During phase II activity or after feeding, slightly less than 50% of all contractions were segmentatory with the remainder propagating over short distances of less than 10 cm. During phase III, on the otherhand, the majority (72%) of contractions propagated and 50% of these travelled for more than 20 cm before petering out. Thus, even during intense activity, contractions propagate over relatively short distances. If peristaltic contractions swept along the whole small bowel the transit would be too fast to allow adequate digestion and absorption of nutrients.

Manometric recordings from perfused catheters placed in the small intestinal lumen reveal tonal changes in addition to the phasic changes reflecting segmentation and peristalsis. These changes in baseline pressure often have phasic contractions superimposed and reflect long-lasting changes in luminal diameter which will also have an effect on the flow of intestinal contents.

A reversal of the net aboral movement of luminal contents can occur shortly before vomiting. The intestine becomes initially quiet before an antiperistaltic contraction sweeps the proximal intestine. The contraction reaches the duodenum just prior to vomiting which expels the gastric contents.

The net effect of all contractile activity is the mixing and aboral progression of digesta with the temporal and spatial relationship between contractions of greater importance than the amplitude of individual waves (Weisbrodt, 1981). The overall rate of progression is referred to as the transit time which decreases with the changing volume and composition of intestinal contents on passage along the intestines. Transit experiments measure the movement of non-absorbable markers or dyes either ingested along with a meal or infused directly into the proximal small intestine. One method of particular clinical use involves the use of unabsorbable sugars (for example, raffinose and stachyose which are abundant in baked beans) as markers of intestinal transit. When the sugars reach the caecum they are degraded by the bacteria in this region and release hydrogen gas as one of the products. This passes through the caecal mucosa into the bloodstream and on to the lungs where it can be detected in the expired air. A rise in the breath hydrogen level marks the arrival of the marker in the caecum (Figure 7.4).

Intraluminal markers have the advantage over ingested markers because they allow propulsion to be estimated during fasting as well as in the fed state. In both man and dog, flow is slowest during phase I and fastest in phase III where peristaltic contractions predominate (Code and Schlegel, 1974; Vantrappen et al., 1977). Bueno, Fioramonti and Ruckebusch (1975) suggested that the greatest rate of propulsion occurred just before phase III with the phase III contractions shutting off the gut orally to the area of propulsion and thus preventing reflux. In animals whose intestinal motility follows the MMC pattern even after feeding, intestinal contents are passed along the small intestine in batches. In animals where the MMC is interrupted by feeding, high rates of flow occur during the fed motor pattern which resembles the phase II activity, consisting of irregular contractions.

Transit is very much faster in the proximal small intestine. Chyme leaving the stomach is very quickly spread over a large area of the duodenum and jejunum to optimize digestion and absorption. A bolus of non-absorbable isotope injected into the upper small intestine takes only 20 min to traverse 50% of the rat small bowel, while the next 30% is covered only after 1 hour (Summers et al., 1970).

This difference in transit time in proximal and distal regions may be due to the higher viscosity of luminal contents in the distal small intestine, because the frequency of contractions is lower distally (see p. 119) or because the velocity at which contractions propagate is less. An alternative explanation may be as a consequence of a pattern of contractions seen only

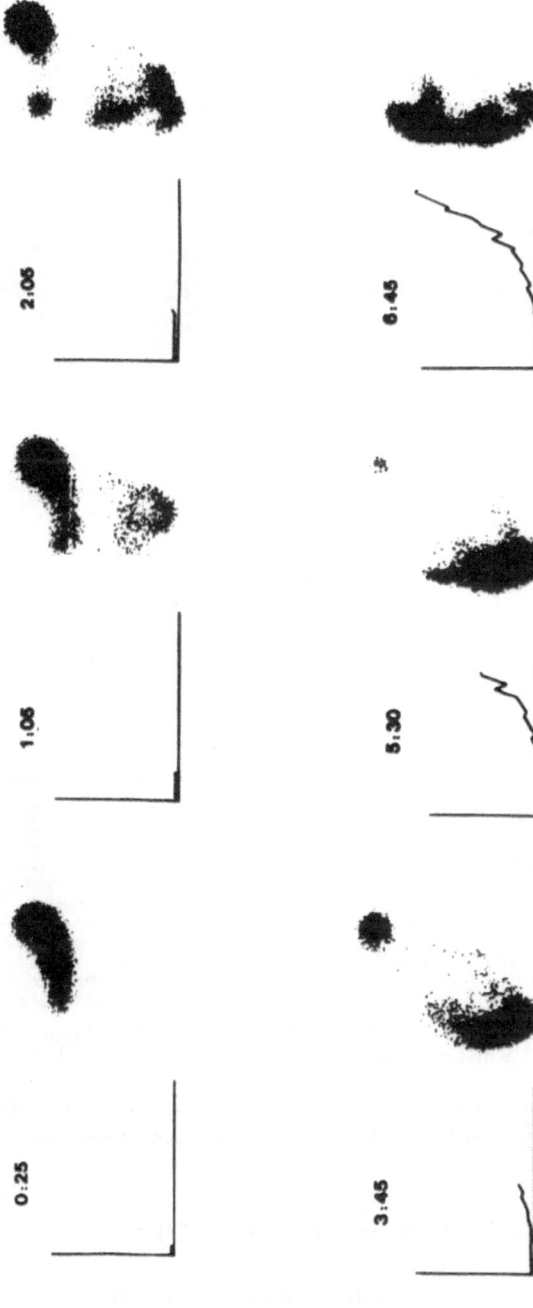

Figure 7.4 Gastrointestinal transit of a single solid meal labelled with technetium-99. On the right of each figure are the gamma camera scans of the abdomen, demonstrating the distribution of the isotope within the gastrointestinal tract. The graph on the left of each figure outlines the breath hydrogen profile up to the time at which the scan was obtained. This time is also shown in hours and minutes above the graph. Note that the initial rise in breath hydrogen corresponded to the apparent entry of radioactivity to the caecum and that the peak hydrogen occurred when almost all of the meal residues were outlining the colon (From Cann and Read, 1981, with kind permission of the authors and publisher, Janssen Pharmaceutical Ltd.)

in the proximal intestine. In the jejunum, during both the fed state and during phase II of the fasted state, contractions are grouped into bursts of about 1 min duration separated by quiescent periods of similar duration. This pattern has therefore been termed the 'minute rhythm' and is suggested to be a major propulsive force in this region (Fleckenstein et al., 1982). Jejunal motility in the anaesthetized ferret shows prominent minute

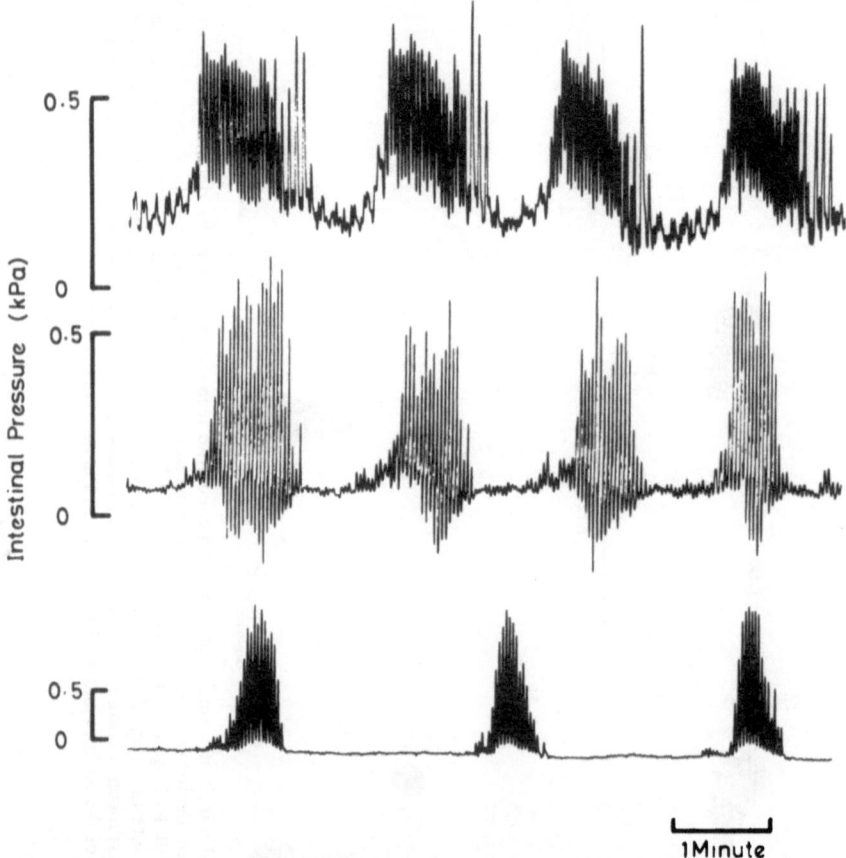

Figure 7.5 Jejunal 'minute rhythms' recorded in three separate animals (From Collman, Grundy and Scratcherd, 1983, with kind permission of the the the editor of J. Physiol. (London))

rhythms (Figure 7.5) and has proved a useful model for the investigation of the mechanisms responsible for their generation (see below, p. 123).

FREQUENCY GRADIENT OF INTESTINAL MOTILITY

A gradient in frequency of contraction along the length of the small intestine has long been recognized. Alvarez (1939) describes examples from several species where the frequency of contraction is highest in the duodenum and lowest in the terminal ileum. A corresponding gradient in slow wave frequency has been confirmed many times. In the small intestine the longitudinal muscle layer is the source of the slow wave which spreads into the circular muscle where it appears to be amplified. These spontaneous oscillations in the resting membrane potential determine the temporal contraction sequence at a given locus. When each slow wave has spikes superimposed upon it, as during phase III of the MMC, the contractions occur at the maximum frequency which is the frequency of the slow waves. At other times the contractions are less regular, for example during phase II or after feeding, when the interval between successive contractions is a multiple of the interval between slow waves. In man the maximal duodenal frequency is $12 \, \text{cycles min}^{-1}$ and $7\text{--}9 \, \text{cycles min}^{-1}$ in the ileum. The dog shows a similar gradient but with a duodenal slow wave frequency of approximately $18 \, \text{cycles min}^{-1}$.

Since adjacent smooth muscle cells are electrotonically coupled, current flows outwards from actively depolarized cells. In the circular muscle layer this coupling ensures that contractions occur almost simultaneously in a circumferential direction. Coupling in the longitudinal muscle layer, however, is a means whereby slow waves in one region can influence those in another. Extracellular recordings from electrodes placed close together on the serosal surface detect slow waves which occur at all points but with a phase lag such that they appear to propagate from a point just below the pylorus, the duodenal pacemaker. The frequency gradient from duodenum to ileum ensures that only propagation in the aboral direction is effective. There is also a gradient in the velocity of propagation being higher in more proximal regions.

The slow wave at one locus influences the occurrence of slow waves in neighbouring regions. If this influence extended the full length of the small intestine there would be no frequency gradient; all regions would contract at the same frequency. However, since this is not the case there must be a limit to how far the dominant frequency can spread. To investigate this point, Diamant and Bortoff (1969) measured the slow wave frequency at short intervals along the whole length of the small intestine of cat, dog and monkey. Instead of a linear decline in slow wave frequency from proximal to distal regions they found that the frequency decreased in a series of steps (Figure 7.6). Long segments of small intestine had the same slow wave frequency with the length of individual plateaux becoming progressively shorter distally. Indeed the first plateau, starting in the duodenum, is variably reported to extend from a third to a half of the total small intestine. At the points between plateaux the waveform detected with the serosal electrodes showed a complex pattern of waxing and waning suggesting interference resulting from two separate slow wave frequencies.

Transection of the intestine at any point results in a marked reduction

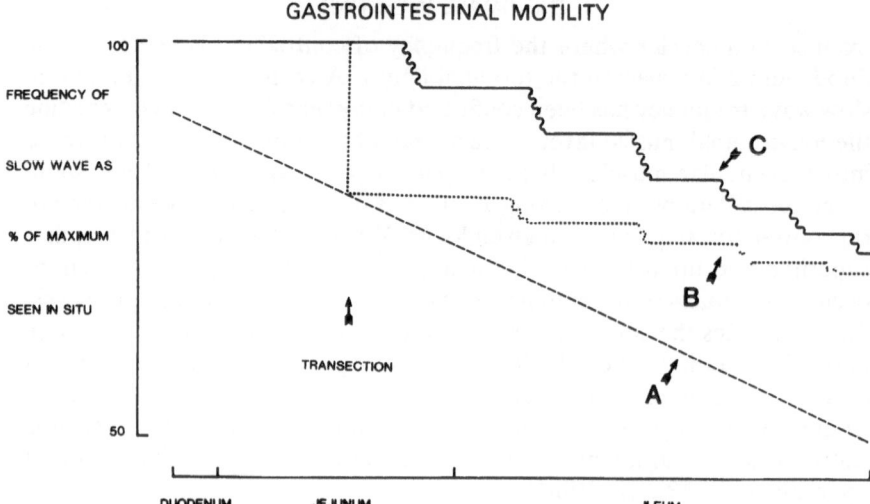

GASTROINTESTINAL MOTILITY

Figure 7.6 Slow wave frequency gradient in the small intestine. **A**: A linear gradient in intrinsic slow wave frequency is seen in segments of intestine removed from various levels of intestine. *In situ* (**C**) the frequency falls in a series of steps. If the intestine is transected at the point indicated, the frequency immediatly distal to the cut falls to that of the intrinsic slow wave frequency (**B**) (Adapted from Diamant and Bortoff, 1969)

in slow wave frequency below the level of transection which in some cases can fall to less than the lowest frequency seen in the terminal ileum prior to transection (see Figure 7.6). When the small intestine is transected into many small sections, or if strips of intestine are removed from various levels along the intestine, a linear gradient in slow wave frequency is seen. Each segment, therefore, has its own intrinsic slow wave frequency but *in situ* this frequency is elevated along the entire length of small intestine.

The explanation of these findings is based on the interaction of a series of oscillators with successively lower intrinsic frequencies which are electrically coupled. Mathematically these are referred to as 'relaxation oscillators', a type of non-linear oscillator that when coupled allow changes in frequency without major changes in waveform. Two neighbouring oscillators, or a series of such oscillators with progressively lower frequencies, will interact by providing an electrical input to the oscillator with the lower frequency. This input would raise the potential of the second, shortening the time to rise to threshold and consequently raise the frequency of the follower to that of the driver. Whether or not one oscillator can drive another depends on the degree of coupling and the difference in frequency. If the frequency of the follower can oscillate at the same frequency as the driver then the two will be entrained and, in the case of the small intestine, a frequency plateau results.

If the difference in intrinsic frequency is too great, or if the coupling is weaker, then the second oscillator is no longer able to follow at the higher frequency and so generates a new, lower frequency. This, however, is not as low as the actual intrinsic slow wave frequency of that region because the input current shortens the interval between some slow waves which are near threshold. The result is that the frequency of the follower is pulled up. Frequency pulling accounts for the higher slow wave frequency *in situ* at all points compared to the intrinsic frequency. It also explains why transection at several levels results in a decrease in frequency distal to each cut.

Computer modelling on the basis of coupled relaxation oscillators give essentially the same characteristics as the *in situ* frequency gradient. One point, however, that could not be accounted for in the computer model and that remains unresolved is the mechanism responsible for the frequency in the initial plateau which is higher than the intrinsic frequency of the highest slow wave oscillator found in the duodenum (see Figure 7.6).

EXTRINSIC NERVOUS CONTROL OF SMALL INTESTINAL MOTILITY

The myogenic properties of intestinal smooth muscle and its regulation by the enteric nervous system has been dealt with previously (see Chapters 1 and 2). The extrinsic parasympathetic and sympathetic innervation modulate these local regulatory mechanisms by firstly providing a background of neural tone that sets the 'basal' level of motility. The basal motility, however, is not a constant baseline of minimal activity but can vary from complete inactivity to intense contractions of maximal amplitude as seen during the activity front of the MMC. The second function of the autonomic nerves is to provide both afferent and efferent pathways for the variety of reflexes which match the small intestinal motility to the biological needs at any particular time. The stimuli that evoke these reflexes usually arise within the wall of the intestine and activate receptor mechanisms in the mucosal, muscle and serosal layers (see Chapter 3). Extraluminal stimuli applied during abdominal surgery, for example, may also activate autonomic reflexes that inhibit intestinal motility leading to paralytic ileus.

The effects of electrical stimulation of the vagal and splanchnic nerves clearly indicate a powerful influence on intestinal motility. The sympathetic innervation is predominantly inhibitory to intestinal motor function via release of noradrenaline. Excitatory effects are mediated mainly via the vagal parasympathetic supply with acetylcholine as the postganglionic transmitter. However, both non-adrenergic, non-cholinergic excitatory and inhibitory effects may also be evoked by stimulation of the vagus after cholinergic blockade. Bayliss and Starling's (1899) initial experiments on the control of small intestinal motility showed a biphasic response to electrical stimulation of the vagus nerve with inhibition followed by excitation. Since atropine was present throughout these experiments the responses represent non-cholinergic phenomena which have subsequently been interpreted as representing inhibition followed by a rebound contraction (see p. 65). However, non-adrenergic, non-cholinergic excitatory transmitter mechanisms have been indicated from *in vitro* studies and recently shown to be activated from a vagal preganglionic input (Collman, Grundy and Scratcherd, 1983).

In the absence of atropine, vagal stimulation in many different species results in powerful excitatory responses mediated via acetylcholine. If the intestine is quiescent, vagal stimulation initiates contractile activity, but if the intestine is spontaneously active, stimulation results in contractions of larger amplitude, and in some cases partial fusion of individual contractions, to give a sustained contraction.

The stimulation of the sympathetic innervation results in inhibition of intestinal motility via the release of noradrenaline from the postganglionic endings. However, as discussed in Chapter 4, the noradrenaline has actions within the myenteric plexus, modifying transmission in the cholinergic pathway, in addition to any direct effects on the smooth muscle.

Stimulation experiments unfortunately give little indication of the role of the parasympathetic and sympathetic innervation in normal regulation but merely show that a particular pathway exists which can produce profound effects when all the fibres in a nerve are simultaneously activated. A more physiological role would be indicated if motility was disrupted following removal of the sympathetic or parasympathetic supply either by nerve section or pharmacological manipulation.

From acute experiments on a variety of different species there is strong evidence for the sympathetic innervation exerting tonic inhibitory influences on intestinal motility. Following sympathetic blockade, strong intestinal contractions could be evoked by electrical vagal stimulation where previously no response or only weak contractions could be elicited. In this type of experiment, therefore, tonic sympathetic activity suppressed the response to vagal stimulation. In acutely prepared, anaesthetized animals some of this sympathetic activity could be attributed to the previous surgery. However, even in chronically prepared animals, section of the splanchnic nerves, removal of the coeliac ganglion or treatment with guanethidine all result in an increase in the level of motility in fasted animals. These results suggest that the sympathetic nerves normally act as a 'brake' on intestinal motility.

In contrast, most studies on the the effect of vagal section would indicate little tonic influence in both acute and chronic animals. Recent studies, however, would appear to be at variance with this conclusion especially where motility in the proximal intestine is concerned. Long-term experiments on vagotomized animals can only be performed after full recovery from the surgery. The relatively normal motility patterns observed under these conditions may, therefore, reflect adaptive changes during the recovery period which allow the enteric nervous system to restore the status quo. A technique has therefore been developed which allows the immediate effects of temporary removal of vagal activity to be studied. Nerve block is achieved by cooling the cervical vagus nerves, which have been previously exteriorized into skin loops, to a temperatures at which conduction ceases (4 °C) while nervous conduction is restored when the vagi are rewarmed. Experiments of this kind indicate that phase II activity in the jejunum of the fasted dog depends on vagal integrity while vagal cooling in the fed animal causes the motility to revert from a fed pattern to one showing cyclical MMC activity (Diamant *et al.*, 1980). The vagus nerves are, therefore, implicated in the disruption of the MMC by feeding (see Chapter 10) and also determine the level of motility in the fed and fasted state.

A similar dependence on an intact vagus has been reported in acute experiments. Jejunal motility in the anaesthetized ferret is organized into 'minute rhythms' that are a characteristic of motility in phase II of the MMC and following feeding. Acute vagal section, atropine or vagal cooling all result in the complete abolition of spontaneous jejunal motility (Figure 7.7).

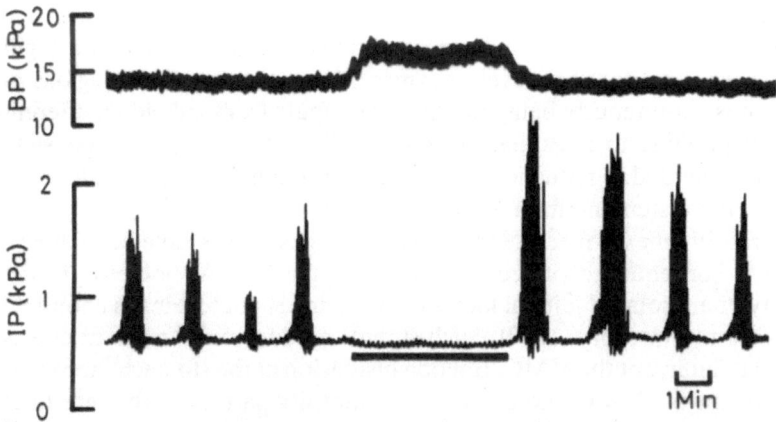

Figure 7.7 The effect of cooling the vagus nerves to below 4 °C (indicated by bar) on jejunal motility (lower trace) and blood pressure (upper trace). The rise in blood pressure marks the period of effective vagal blockade during which time jejunal 'minute rhythms' are abolished (From Collman, Grundy and Scratcherd, 1983, with kind permission of the the the editor of J. Physiol. (London))

Motility in the ileum is less dependent on its vagal innervation. In the anaesthetized ferret there is a gradation in the disruptive effect of vagal section, vagal cooling and atropine, with these procedures abolishing jejunal motility but having relatively little effect on the ileum (Collman, Grundy and Scratcherd, 1984b). This observation fits well with histological data which demonstrates a gradual reduction in the number of vagal fibres projecting to progressively distal segments of small intestine.

It would seem reasonable to conclude, therefore, that the level of intestinal motility, especially in proximal regions, is dependent on the balance between activity in the vagal and splanchnic nerve supply. The actual amount of tonic activity in the different divisions of the efferent supply will be modified by the impulse traffic in the afferent fibres making synaptic contact with them. Reflex control of intestinal motility is therefore mediated by alterations in the balance of the parasympathetic and sympathetic activity which results specifically in either enhanced or reduced intestinal motility.

Of all intestinal reflexes the best characterized is the intestinointestinal inhibitory reflex elicited by distension of the bowel wall. The pathway for this reflex is sympathetic and mediated through the release of noradrenaline, but there is some debate as to the relative importance of the spinal cord and prevertebral ganglia as the reflex centre responsible (see p. 49). The reflex is activated by distension of the intestine which, if the stimulus is powerful enough, results in inhibition of the whole gastrointestinal tract. Such stimuli are likely to arise under pathophysiological conditions, for example bowel obstruction or after abdominal surgery when manipulation of the bowel results in paralytic ileus. However, reflex suppression of intestinal motility can occur with only small distending volumes generating pressures less than those seen during spontaneous contractions. One might argue, therefore, that the level of sympathetic tone to various regions of intestine is continuously being modified by inputs from individual afferent fibres responding to intestinal movement. Should a segment of intestine become distended, a reduction in motility in proximal regions would allow time for the distending fluid to be dispersed.

Excitatory reflexes mediated through the vagus nerves have been described as a consequence of feeding (see Chapter 10). An increase in the motility of an isolated jejunal loop in dog during sham feeding is abolished by vagotomy (Gregory, 1950). Such stimuli produce only transient effects and fail to interrupt the MMC. Balloon distension of the stomach, however, does disrupt the MMC and evokes a fed motility pattern in the intestines but is less effective than a nutrient meal. Since both responses are impaired by vagotomy the response would appear to be nerve mediated and constitute a gastrointestinal reflex.

HORMONAL CONTROL OF SMALL INTESTINAL MOTILITY

Many of the gastrointestinal hormones affect small intestinal motility. A role for a variety of these in the regulation of the MMC and its disruption by feeding are discussed in Chapters 9 and 10. In general, gastrin, CCK and motilin stimulate contractions while secretin, glucagon, VIP and GIP inhibit motor activity. However, whether the response to these hormones represents a physiological mechanism of control is yet to be determined. In this respect CCK is probably the most important because the blood levels required to stimulate pancreatic secretion and gallbladder contractions also stimulate intestinal motility. Part of this action involves the release of acetylcholine from intramural neurones and illustrates the importance of interactions between neural and hormonal mechanisms. Interactions between different hormones are also likely to be important. Secretin, for example, seldom inhibits spontaneous intestinal motility but markedly reduces the response to mechanical distension or infusions of gastrin and CCK.

The different balance of hormones released by meals of different composition may be responsible for the variable levels of motility seen in the fed state. The introduction of fat into the terminal ileum causes a marked delay in both gastric emptying and small intestinal transit time. Such a mechanism may rely on the release of hormones from the distal ileum and provide a means of matching transit to luminal composition.

THE ILEOCAECAL SPHINCTER

The ileocaecal sphincter marks the boundary between the small and large intestine. It is an anatomically recognizable structure having thicker musculature than the adjacent ileum and colon, and in man it protrudes into and is surrounded by the wall of the colon. This gives the sphincter a valve-like appearance and serves to ensure one-way traffic from ileum to colon and so limits the entrance of colonic bacteria into the small intestine. In man a 4 cm long region of high pressure can be detected with a resting pressure some 20 mmHg above that in the colon. Colonic distension enhances this pressure in a way that is consistent with a role in preventing reflux from the colon; however, this may be a passive phenomenon because of the junction's valve-like arrangement.

Tone in the sphincter depends mainly on the myogenic properties of the smooth muscle in this region (see Weisbrodt, 1981). Isolated strips of muscle from the cat and opossum have a resting tone which is unaffected by treatment with tetrodotoxin. Activity in the intrinsic and extrinsic nerve supply does, however, modify this tone. An inhibitory nervous influence has been demonstrated by transmural electrical stimulation *in vitro*. On the other hand, only excitatory responses are seen *in vivo*, as indicated by a reduced trans-sphincteric flow, when either the sympathetic or parasympathetic nerves are stimulated (Pahlin and Kewenter, 1976). Like the arrangement in the lower oesophageal sphincter, sympathetic stimulation is mediated via alpha-adrenoreceptors while parasympathetic influences are blocked by atropine.

Distension of the ileum causes sphincter relaxation in both dog and man

125

and may be a prerequisite for the passage of digesta into the colon. Experiments in cats failed to show this relaxation and, interestingly, in these experiments the continuity of the ileum oral to the sphincter had been interrupted (Pahlin and Kewenter, 1975). The relaxation seen in other experiments may therefore represent a descending wave of inhibition associated with a peristaltic reflex evoked by the distension. As such the propagation of the peristaltic wave into the sphincter would force intestinal contents ahead of it and on into the colon. Such an interpretation would account for the observation that inhibitory responses are seen only when the intramural nerves are stimulated and not during stimulation of the extrinsic supply.

The continuity of the bowel wall is lost at the ileocaecal sphincter. This ensures a barrier for transmission and allows completely independent motility in the two adjacent regions. The ileum shows MMC activity while the caecum does not. As will be seen in the next chapter, this arrangement is essential for the normal functioning of the large intestine.

8
The large intestine

INTRODUCTION

The large intestine can be divided on the basis of its motor function into two separate regions. The proximal region consisting of caecum and ascending colon serves a reservoir function while more distal regions are important for the periodic elimination of faecal waste. Herbivores, especially those of the horse and rabbit family, derive considerable nutrient from the bacterial breakdown of plant fibre within the caecum. In these species, therefore, the caecum is enlarged and more complex than in the carnivore, whose digestive processes are more or less complete before the digesta leaves the ileum, so consequently the carnivore colon is short and simple.

The large intestine of man shows characteristics of both herbivore and carnivore. It is haustrated like that of most herbivores but relatively short (about 1.5 meters in length) compared to the rest of the bowel. About 500 ml of digesta, consisting of a mixture of water and indigestible vegetable fibre, enters the caecum each day. During its stay here bacterial fermentation releases nutrients that are absorbed, along with much of the water and electrolytes, so that the volume is reduced and the contents become more solid. These are slow processes requiring a prolonged stay in this region. While it takes only a few hours for ingested material to reach the caecum, its journey through the rest of the large intestine is measured in days.

Contractile activity in more distal regions of the large intestine maintain the slow aboral progression of faecal material. On occasions, however, a small volume of material in the proximal colon is separated from the main mass and moved rapidly through the distal colon. In this way caecal contents are moved long distances and on occasions propelled all the way to the terminal colon in preparation for evacuation. The distal colon therefore plays an excretory role and is responsible for propelling the more solid faecal material into the rectum prior to defaecation.

The motor function of the proximal and distal colon appear to be specifically adapted to their different roles. However, the underlying control mechanisms have not been resolved to the extent of those regulating motility in the rest of the gastrointestinal tract. In this chapter an overview of large intestinal motility and its control will be presented and where possible related to the human bowel.

ANATOMY OF THE HUMAN LARGE INTESTINE

The large intestine viewed radiographically shows the gross anatomical features that distinguish it from the small intestine (Figure 8.1). It is divided

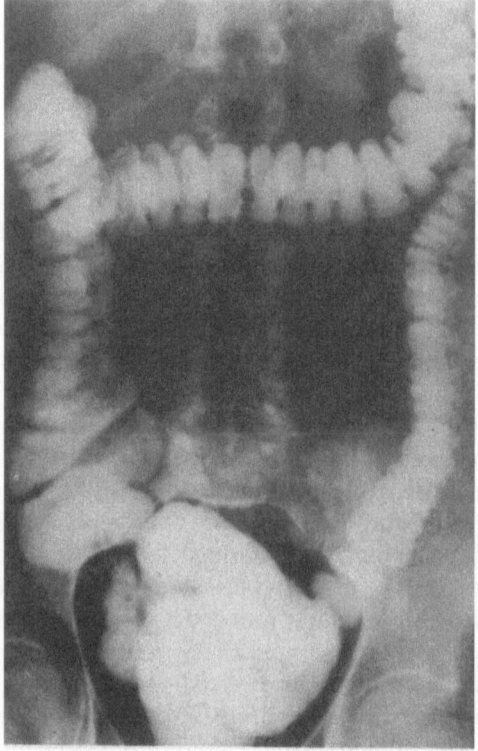

Figure 8.1 Barium enema of the colon. Note the haustrated appearence of the bowel wall (From Sleisenger and Silverberg, 1978, with kind permission of the authors and publisher, W.B. Saunders Co.)

into several regions on the basis of its position within the abdominal cavity. Thus the colon consists of ascending, transverse, and descending segments with the terminal convoluted region of the latter termed the sigmoid colon. The caecum consists of the few centimetres of bowel that lie upstream from the point of entry of the ileum while the most distal segment is the rectum.

The caecum and ascending colon are more dilated than distal regions, and it is this area that plays the reservoir role.

A feature of the colon that is highlighted in radiographic plates is the haustrated appearance of the bowel wall (see Figure 8.1). These haustrations arise because of the specialized arrangement of the longitudinal muscle layer in this region. Whereas the longitudinal muscle is a layer of uniform thickness in the oesophagus, stomach and small intestine, in the colon the muscle fibres are grouped into three parallel bands of muscle (the taeniae coli) separated by a much thinner layer of muscle. These taeniae are normally held at a slightly shorter length than the underlying layers which consequently bulge between the taeniae and also pucker inwards at regular intervals to give the haustrated appearance. These haustra are not rigid structures but disappear and reappear at different locations at different times. However, some haustra are rigid and remain after the taeniae are cut or after death, and these are associated with thickened bands of circular muscle with folding of the underlying mucosa.

Haustrations were originally considered only as a means of increasing the mucosal surface area. However, a motor function 'vital to the comfort and social security of the individual' arises because it increases the resistance to flow from one pocket to the next which slows down transit and provides a more controlled delivery of faeces into the rectum.

MOTOR PATTERNS AND THE FLOW OF DIGESTA

The standard techniques of radiography, manometry and electromyography have allowed the motor activity of the large intestine to be characterized. Unfortunately, however, each approach has generated an array of terminology which essentially describe the same thing, that is movement of the bowel wall, but which are not readily comparable. It is convenient, therefore, to summarize the results of each type of study separately before the control mechanisms are considered.

Motor patterns distinguished radiographically

Viewed radiographically the colon is seldom totally inactive. Movements of some kind are always present somewhere in the colon. These movements are generally associated with contractions of individual haustra, or several haustra simultaneously, and segmentary in nature. A reduction in diameter of one haustra will displace contents in both directions thereby churning the contents while simultaneously reducing net transit. However, the sequential contraction of adjacent haustra in either direction cause propulsion or retropulsion of luminal contents. In the proximal colon contractions generally migrate orally while in the distal colon the direction of propagation is aboral. In one of the earliest studies of this kind, Cannon (1902) described the contraction sequence in the conscious cat. 'Antiperistaltic contraction' occurred intermittently in the proximal colon. During a burst of activity, contractions were generated at a frequency of 5–6 min^{-1} and travelled orally at 1–2 mm s^{-1} down the ascending colon. This region has been confirmed as the major site for delay in transit through the bowel of healthy human volunteers. These 'guinea-pigs' ingested three different-sized radio-opaque discs with each of three meals taken 36, 24 and 12 hours before X-ray examination. A 12-hour gap would ensure that the contents of one meal would have entered the caecum before the next was ingested. Yet the discs were found to be freely mixed throughout the colon with some of the most recently ingested discs lying ahead of some that had been eaten the day before (Halls, 1965).

Thus in the proximal colon segmentary contractions have a tendency to propagate orally and so retain and mix the intestinal contents. In the transverse and descending colon, segmenting contractions generally propagate aborally ensuring that the contents are propelled slowly towards the rectum. True peristaltic contractions, which by definition are preceded by a descending wave of relaxation, are a relatively rare event compared to the slowly migrating haustral contractions. However, a much more effective propulsive force, seen to occur only a few times per day and more commonly after a meal, has been termed a 'mass movement'. These movements have several characteristics when seen radiographically. The event is marked initially by the disappearance of haustral folds over a length of colon. A contraction then starts at the proximal end of that segment and moves rapidly caudally propelling an entire segment of faecal material into the distal colon and rectum. The haustral folds return and segmenting waves resume.

Distension of the rectum generally gives rise to the urge to defaecate. Alvarez (1939) describes the case of a man with an incompetent anus who suffered the urge to defaecate each time a mass movement occurred. He had a call soon after getting out of bed, another when he began breakfast and one or two more following the meal: 'After that, in order to save himself trouble, he had to avoid the sight, smell or even thought of food, so in walking down the street he was careful not to pass in front of restaurants. A few of his friends, knowing his weakness, sometimes amused themselves by discussing before him the relative merits of Hungarian goulash and beefsteak and onions.'

Manometric recordings of colonic motility

Recordings from intraluminal balloons, perfused catheters and radiotelemetric devices, or from extraluminal strain gauges, distinguish only three types of contractile event which may be surprising given the repertoire of movements described radiographically. However, in studies combining the two techniques it has been noted that considerable flow could occur with little pressure variations and, vice versa, large pressure waves without significant flow. In this respect, therefore, it is the temporal and spatial relationship of contractions that is important and not the amplitude and waveform of individual contractions. Nevertheless, as a method of quantifying colonic motor activity for investigations of the control mechanisms, pressure manometry or extraluminal strain gauge recordings provide useful data, especially when a series of such recording devices allow the direction and distance of propagation of contractions to be quantified.

The original classification of pressure waves in the dog colon by Templeton and Lawson (1931) distinguished low-amplitude, short-duration contractions (type I) from longer-duration, high-amplitude contractions (type II). In addition type III waves were long-lasting changes in baseline tone which probably reflect changes in luminal diameter. Similar types of contraction have repeatedly been observed in man. Waves corresponding to type I contractions have been reported with frequencies varying from 5 to 13 min^{-1} and intraluminal pressure rises of less than 1 kPa. Waves similar to type II contractions have a duration of 12–60 s and generate pressures greater than 10 kPa. These latter frequently occur in bursts which can either be stationary or migrate in either direction.

Electrical correlates of colonic activity

Colonic smooth muscle generates slow waves and spikes. Like the small intestine, slow waves determine the temporal arrangement of contractions which occur when spiking activity is superimposed on the peak of the slow wave. However, the slow waves recorded from colonic muscle originate in the circular muscle layer and generally occur at a lower frequency than those in the small intestine. In the isolated whole cat colon *in vitro* the frequency of slow waves in the proximal colon were marginally lower, at 4.5 cycles min^{-1}, than that in the distal colon, 6 cycles min^{-1}. This reversal in frequency gradient from that seen in the small intestine would, by analogy, account for the presence of orally directed contractions seen predominantly in the proximal regions. A pacemaker zone in the mid colon was demonstrated by sectioning the colon at several levels. After transection, the slow wave frequency in the proximal colon became even lower and the frequency gradient to the mid colonic pacemaker steeper. However, the slow wave frequency over the mid and distal region of colon showed little if any gradient and was relatively unaffected by transection (Christensen, Anuras and Hauser, 1974). The shallowness of the gradient in the distal colon, and the poorer coupling that appeared to exist between neighbouring regions, would ensure that the slow waves spread only over short distances but could do so in either direction.

Electrical recordings from the human distal colon have been made using probes, inserted through the anus, which are either clipped to the mucosa or held in place by suction. Such recordings raise two problems. First, the slow wave is not omnipresent but appears intermittently for between 5 and 85% of the total recording time depending on the study; and second, when the slow wave is present it shows an extremely variable frequency (see Christensen, 1981). Computer analysis of such records detect several (usually two) independent slow wave frequencies. The latter could be due to poor coupling between smooth muscle cells as indicated by the lack of spread of slow waves along the bowel. Thus, a single recording electrode, especially when it is attached to the mucosa and therefore at a distance from the circular muscle layer, may simultaneously detect slow waves generated by several different bundles of smooth muscle.

The intermittency of the slow wave is another controversial point. It could be an artifact caused by intermittent contact between the recording electrode and the mucosal surface. Alternatively, it may be a real phenomenon reflecting a species difference between man and cats and dogs which do show an omnipresent slow wave. Such a difference is indicated from *in vitro* recordings of colonic slow waves where good contact is ensured but intermittent slow waves are still observed. In other species (rabbit and pig) intermittent slow waves have also been reported.

Spiking activity superimposed on the slow waves generates muscle contractions and the recording of these spikes from the serosal or mucosal surface is often used as an index of contractile activity. Two types of spiking activity have been described (Figure 8.2). Spikes occurring during a single slow wave are referred to as short spike bursts (SSB) (Ruckebusch and Fioramonti, 1980) or discrete electrical response activity (DERA) (Sarna et al., 1981b). These short spike bursts occur at the slow wave frequency and do not migrate, properties reminiscent of type I pressure waves. The second type of spike burst is not related to the slow wave frequency and can actually extend through several slow wave cycles. These long spike bursts (LSB) or continuous electrical response activity (CERA) can migrate in either direction or be stationary, and are therefore electrical correlates of type II pressure waves. A third electrical event not associated with spiking activity has been described as the contractile electrical complex (CEC). These are rapidly oscillating potentials superimposed on the slow wave which migrate and induce contractions which persist for the duration of the oscillations. These may be electrical correlates of mass movements.

Physiological significance of colonic contractions

In an attempt to understand exactly how the colon moves faecal material, many research workers have tried to correlate flow studies with manometry, manometry with electromyography, and electromyography with flow. As

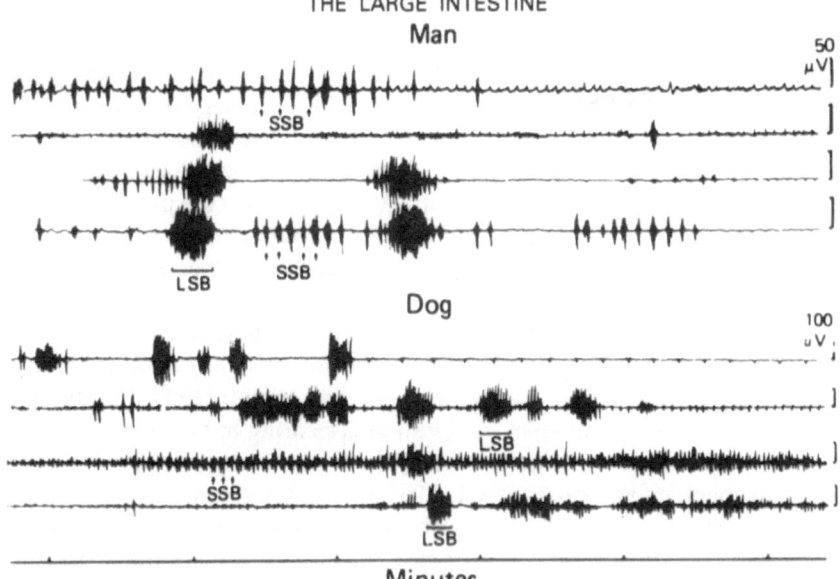

THE LARGE INTESTINE

Figure 8.2 Electrical activity in the colon of man and dog both exhibiting short (SSB) and long spike bursts (LSB). In man, the electrical activity was recorded from an intraluminal probe with four electrodes spaced 10 cm apart in the descending colon. In the dog, recordings were made with chronically implanted serosal electrodes also 10 cm apart beginning 5 cm from the ileo-colonic junction (From Bueno and Fioramonti, 1981, with kind permission of the authors and publisher, Janssen Pharmaceutical Ltd.)

mentioned above, the effect of colonic contractions on flow of contents depends not so much on the waveform of contractions but on the degree and direction of propagation and the kind of activity that precedes or follows. In general, short-duration, low-amplitude contractions are stationary while 'long-duration, large-amplitude contractions are progressive. Electromyographic studies correlate well with pressure waves or strain gauge recordings. Waves of short duration at the slow wave frequency are associated with short spike bursts on each slow wave. Long-duration contractions correlate with long spike bursts which migrate both orally and aborally. Some long spike bursts do not migrate and these produce long-duration localized contractions. These different patterns of activity are sufficient to account for all the observations on colonic movement described radiographically.

A recent study by Ehrlein, Reich and Schwinger (1982) came to similar conclusions from consideration of pressure waves and cineradiography in the rabbit colon. The contractions with the highest frequency were associated with 'rolling movements of the haustra' which were suggested to represent the antiperistaltic waves described in earlier studies. Segmental activity, which divided up the colonic contents, was seen as persistent rings of contraction which migrated aborally at approximately $7\,\mathrm{mm\,s^{-1}}$. The

133

pressure correlate of these waves were slow rises in baseline pressure of several minutes' duration. True peristaltic contractions appeared as monophasic pressure waves of 10 s duration which propagated at $13\,\mathrm{mm\,s^{-1}}$. These occurred only once or twice per hour and were associated with the disappearance of segmental activity distally. These are characteristics of the mass movements described in man, although in man the pressure waves are of longer duration and propagate at only $5\,\mathrm{mm\,s^{-1}}$.

It would appear, therefore, that even given the enormous species variations in colonic structure, the motor pattern shows essentially the same features with frequent short and long-duration contractions and the occasional mass movement. In six different species, including man, examined in a comparative study by Ruckebusch and Fioramonti (1980), all showed short spike bursts of less than 5 s duration appearing in bursts of localized activity lasting several minutes. Long spike bursts occurred individually or grouped together and propagated. Mixing of colonic contents was linked to short spike burst activity while propulsion occurred during long spike burst activity; the overall rate of propulsion being determined by the proportion of time occupied by the latter (Figure 8.3). Disturbances of

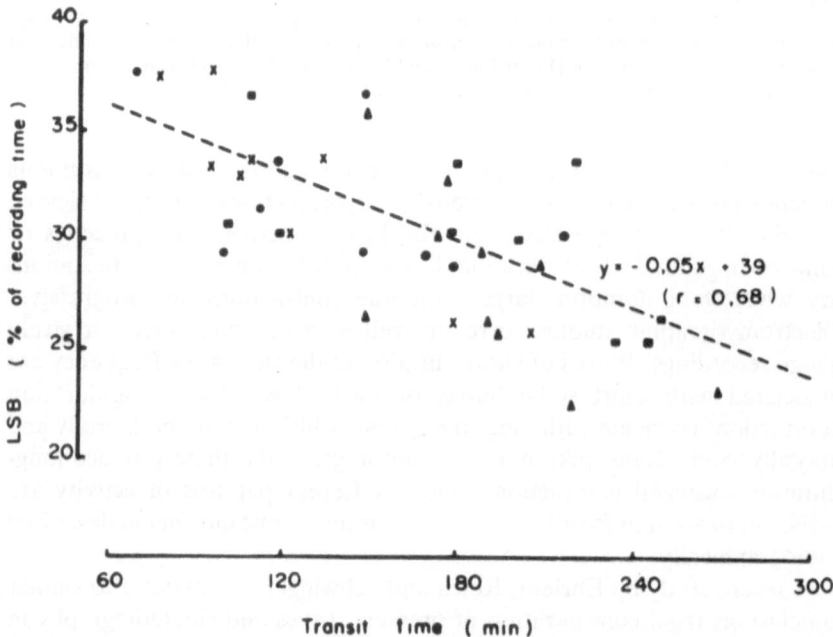

Figure 8.3 Relationship between colonic transit time determined by the movement of an unabsorbable marker along a 30 cm segment of canine proximal colon and the percentage of the recording time occupied by long spike bursts (LSB). Each value corresponded to a single experiment performed in different dogs designated by individual symbols (From Bueno and Fioramonti, 1981, with kind permission of the authors and publisher, Janssen Pharmaceutical Ltd.)

colonic motility resulting in constipation or diarrhoea may be associated with an alteration in the ratio of long and short spike bursts (Bueno *et al.*, 1980).

CONTROL OF LARGE INTESTINAL MOTILITY

Intrinsic nervous control

The enteric nervous system in the colon has not been systematically studied to the extent of that in the small intestine. However, there is every reason to believe that a similar arrangement of intramural connections exists within the wall of the colon. The cat colon *in vitro* is continuously suppressed by tonic neural elements in the intramural plexuses. Thus, treatment with tetrodotoxin or local anaesthetic results in excitation of the circular muscle layer. Also, congenital agangliosis of the colonic wall (Hirschsprung's disease) is associated with a zone of circular muscle spasm. Contractions of the circular muscle may therefore partly result from the periodic removal of this tonic inhibition.

A second indicator of similar controls in the small and large intestine is the presence of intramural pathways mediating ascending excitation and descending inhibition during activation of the peristaltic reflex. This was examined in detail by Costa and Furness (1976) in isolated segments of guinea-pig colon. Stretching the wall of the colon resulted in the development of a contraction above the point of stimulation while relaxation was evident for several centimetres below the point of stretch. Interruption of Auerbach's plexus abolished these effects with the descending inhibition being mediated by a non-adrenergic, non-cholinergic transmitter.

Transmural electrical stimulation illustrates this motor innervation since both excitatory and inhibitory response can be evoked. The excitatory response involves both cholinergic and non-cholinergic transmitters while the inhibitory response is non-adrenergic and non-cholinergic.

Extrinsic nervous mechanisms

Parasympathetic influences

The study of the parasympathetic nervous control of colonic motility is complicated by the dual source of this innervation. The vagus nerve provides the parasympathetic supply to the proximal colon while more distal regions receive their parasympathetic innervation from the sacral spinal cord by way of the pelvic nerves. There is no distinct level where one takes over from the other, more a region of considerable overlap with a large part of the colon receiving a supply from both.

Vagal control – Acute and chronic vagal section has generally been reported to have little effect on colonic motility. However, the intramural plexuses together with the supply from the pelvic nerves may be able to adapt to the lack of a vagal input. Recent studies on colonic motility in the anaesthetized ferret indicate considerable vagal influence on proximal colonic motility (Collman, Grundy and Scratcherd, 1984a). In these experiments a reversible vagotomy was achieved by cooling the cervical vagus nerves; a procedure which caused a marked reduction in colonic motility (Figure 8.4).

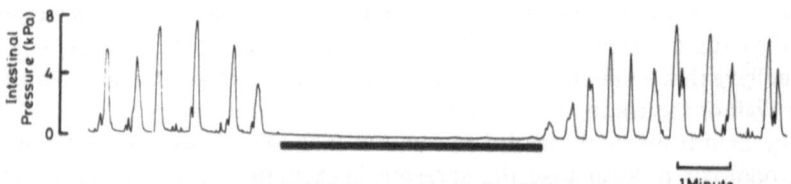

Figure 8.4 The effect of vagal cooling on spontaneous colonic motility. The bar indicates the period in which the nerves were below 4 °C (From Collman, Grundy and Scratcherd, 1984a, with kind permission of the the editor of J. Physiol. (London))

Atropine reduces but does not abolish colonic contractions. In the ferret this atropine-resistant motility is also sensitive to vagal integrity as indicated by its reduction following vagal cooling. These results imply that two excitatory vagal pathways exist, one to cholinergic postganglionic neurones and the other to non-cholinergic neurones – a conclusion consistent with the finding of electrical vagal stimulation which evokes both cholinergic and non-cholinergic contractile responses in ferret, cat and dog. Thus tonic activity in both cholinergic and non-cholinergic pathways contributes to the level of spontaneous motility in the proximal colon. There have been no reports of vagally mediated inhibition of colonic motility.

Pelvic control – The importance of the pelvic nerves is obvious from lesion experiments. Destruction of the sacral parasympathetic pathway markedly depresses colonic contractility. That motility is still present after decentralization suggests that the enteric nervous system can still coordinate propulsive movements even without a parasympathetic supply. However, the sustained propulsive contractions, evoked by colonic and rectal distension, that are associated with defaecation are abolished by section of the pelvic nerves. Nervous activity recorded from the pelvic nerves during rectal distension reveals an efferent discharge that is modulated in phase with colonic contractions with the nervous activity preceding the rise in colonic pressure indicating contractions (Figure 8.5). What these nerve fibres may be doing is illustrated by electrical stimulation of the pelvic nerves. Powerful propulsive contractions can be elicited by such procedures that are mediated by both cholinergic and non-cholinergic mechanisms (Fasth *et al.*, 1980). In addition a non-adrenergic, non-cholinergic inhibitory innervation can be demonstrated to the distal colon which

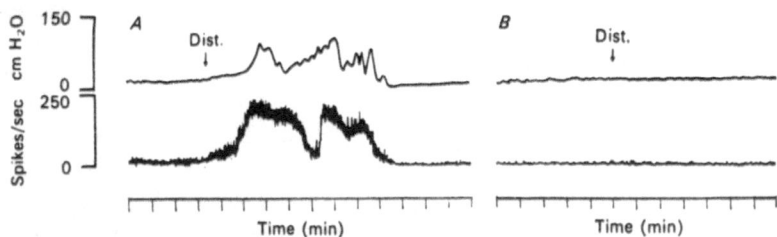

Figure 8.5 Correlation between proximal colonic motility and firing in parasympathetic efferent nerves to the colon following colonic distension in the chloralose anaesthetized cat. The upper trace is intraluminal pressure and the lower trace represents the integrated neural discharge. A: a 2 ml distension evoked a reflex increase in efferent neurone activity and induced colonic contractions which were abolished by sectioning the sacral roots (**B**) (From De Groat and Krier, 1978, with kind permission of the authors and the editor of J. Physiol. (London))

may be involved in the accommodation of faecal material in the rectum and distal colon.

Sympathetic influences

Tonic activity in the sympathetic nerves appears to continuously suppress colonic motor activity. Section of the thoracic or lumbar splanchnic nerves results in an increase in proximal and distal motility respectively. Electrical stimulation, not surprisingly, inhibits contractile activity, reducing both tone and phasic contractions. These effects are mediated via noradrenaline acting predominantly within the enteric nerve plexuses.

Reflex control of colonic motility

Both parasympathetic and sympathetic reflex responses to afferent nerve stimulation have been described but only two reflexes, apart from the defaecation reflex (see p. 140), have received sufficient attention to elucidate any sort of mechanism. The first of these is an extension of the intestinointestinal inhibitory reflex described in the previous chapter. Distension of the proximal colon inhibits motor activity in the distal colon, while distension of the latter inhibits contractions of the former, both via sympathetic reflexes. These colocolonic reflexes can be elicited in the decentralized colon provided that its connections with the prevertebral ganglia are intact. Sectioning the intermesenteric nerves, which connect the inferior mesenteric ganglia with the more proximal coeliac and superior mesenteric ganglia, abolishes the reflexes (Figure 8.6). The reflex is therefore mediated through the prevertebral ganglia with the postganglionic noradrenergic fibres making the link with the intramural plexuses (Kreulen and Szurszewski, 1979).

The second reflex relates to the increase in colonic motility that generally follows a meal. The intake of food is followed by an overall increase in

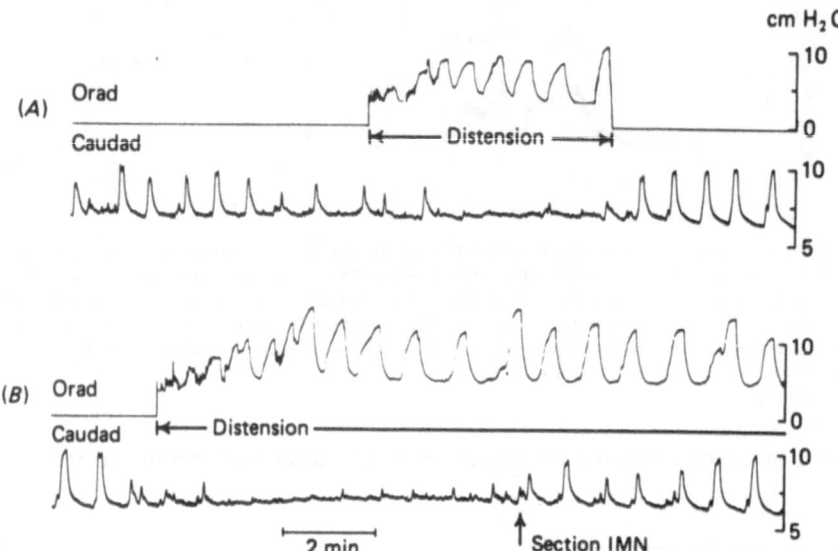

Figure 8.6 Effect of distension of an oral segment of colon on contractions in a caudal segment and the effect of sectioning the intermesenteric nerve (IMN). The intraluminal pressure was zero before and after distension. The trace in **B** begins 2 min after the end of panel **A** (From Kreulen and Szurszewski, 1979, with kind permission of the authors and the editor of J. Physiol. (London))

the number and frequency of contractions in both proximal and distal regions and also an increased likelihood of mass movements, leading to rectal distension and the urge to defaecate. This colonic response to feeding is common knowledge. Mothers with young babies use it as the basis for toilet training while in adults it contributes towards an individual's regular habit.

This generally recognized response to feeding has been termed the gastrocolic reflex. However, as Christensen (1981) pointed out recently 'the response is not clearly established as neural, the stimulus is not confined to the stomach and the response is not confined to the colon'.

Cephalic stimuli have been implicated in mans' colonic response to food as indicated in the example quoted earlier from Alvarez (1939). However, deliberate attempts to establish a colonic motor response to the anticipation of food have failed. This is possibly because of the undoubted fact that the colon is extremely sensitive to emotional states which may alter its responsiveness to extracolonic influences.

The entry of food into the stomach and intestines would therefore seem to be the major stimulus, but the connections between these proximal regions on the one hand and the colon on the other is still to be clearly established. The response can be extremely prompt, with a visible increase in motility only minutes after the ingestion of food implicating a neural component (Snape *et al.*, 1979). Consistent with this is the observation that atropine delays the response to food suggesting an early neural response mediated via acetylcholine reinforced by a slower, and possibly hormonal, non-cholinergic mechanism. The neural pathway could be vagal since section of these nerves abolished the caecal motor response to feeding in the rabbit (Ruckebusch, Grivel and Fargeas, 1971). However, since vagotomy removes both afferent and efferent pathways in the vagus, the loss of the response could be due to removal of one or both of these. The presence of a vagovagal reflex to the colon is evident from electrical stimulation experiments. Stimulating the afferent fibres in one branch of the vagus nerves in the thorax evokes powerful colonic contractions which are abolished when the remaining branches, below the site of stimulation,

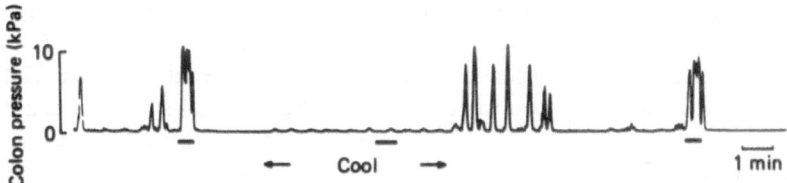

Figure 8.7 The colonic response to central vagal stimulation at 5 Hz before, during, and after cooling the dorsal and ventral vagal trunks to 2 °C. The stimulus period is denoted by bar. Note that vagal cooling completely abolished the response to afferent vagal stimulation (From Collman *et al.*, 1984c, with kind permission of the the editor of J. Physiol. (London))

are cooled to prevent conduction (Figure 8.7). The pathway exists, therefore, but the question is: what activates it?

The stomach is not necessary as a source for the stimulation of colonic motility since motor responses occur in patients who have had complete gastrectomies, and perfusion of loops of intestine with various nutrients can also stimulate colonic motility. There are further difficulties in elucidating the control mechanisms for, on feeding, the terminal ileum is also stimulated. It has been proposed that the colonic response follows indirectly from an increased discharge of intestinal contents into the colon.

Hormonal control

The colon, like the rest of the gastrointestinal tract, responds to many of the gut hormones. However, only gastrin and CCK are believed to play a regulatory role and this in the colonic response to a meal. Both increase motility at doses comparable to the levels found circulating after a meal although the blood concentrations of CCK correlate better with colonic activity than the levels of gastrin. Renny *et al.*, (1983) suggests that the delayed response to feeding after treatment with atropine is mediated through CCK. However, both gastrin and CCK have an action that is in part mediated through the release of acetylcholine which would also be affected by atropine. Thus at present the colonic motor response to eating may be well documented, however, the mechanisms involved are far from resolved.

DEFAECATION

The defaecation reflex is a complex response to distension of the rectum which involves the coordinated activity of the internal and external anal sphincters, the distal colon and the muscles of the pelvic floor, abdominal wall and diaphragm.

The anal sphincters

The internal anal spincter is a thickening of the circular smooth muscle layer 2.5–3 cm long at the terminal part of the rectum. The external anal sphincter is a striated muscle which surrounds the internal sphincter. Both sphincters are tonically contracted but only the external sphincter can be subjected to voluntary control. Being a striated muscle, the external anal sphincter is under neurogenic control. It is maintained closed through tonic activity in its motor innervation from the sacral spinal cord via the pudendal nerve. Since this is its only innervation it follows that relaxation of the sphincter is mediated through suppression of this tonic nervous activity.

Tone in the internal anal sphincter is partly neurogenic. Studies in several species have revealed an excitatory innervation from both cholinergic and noradrenergic nerves with the latter operating through alpha-adrenergic receptors and contributing to the maintained sphincter closure. A non-adrenergic, non-cholinergic inhibitory innervation is also present, and since relaxation of the sphincter is resistant to cholinergic and adrenergic blockade it is presumably responsible for sphincter relaxation. There is still speculation, however, as to whether these inhibitory nerves are activated through spinal reflexes or through descending pathways in the intramural plexuses.

The defaecation reflex

The propulsion of faeces into the rectum by mass movements is the stimulus for defaecation. Mechanoreceptors in the rectum detect the degree of distension and are responsible for initiating the defaecation reflex. However, the sequence of events that follows can be reinforced or suppressed as a consequence of the stimulation of receptors lining the anal canal. These receptors can detect the consistency of faecal matter, and in man are subtly tuned to allow, for example, gas to be passed at times when it would be socially embarrassing to pass anything else.

Responses of the rectum and anal sphincters to rectal distension can be

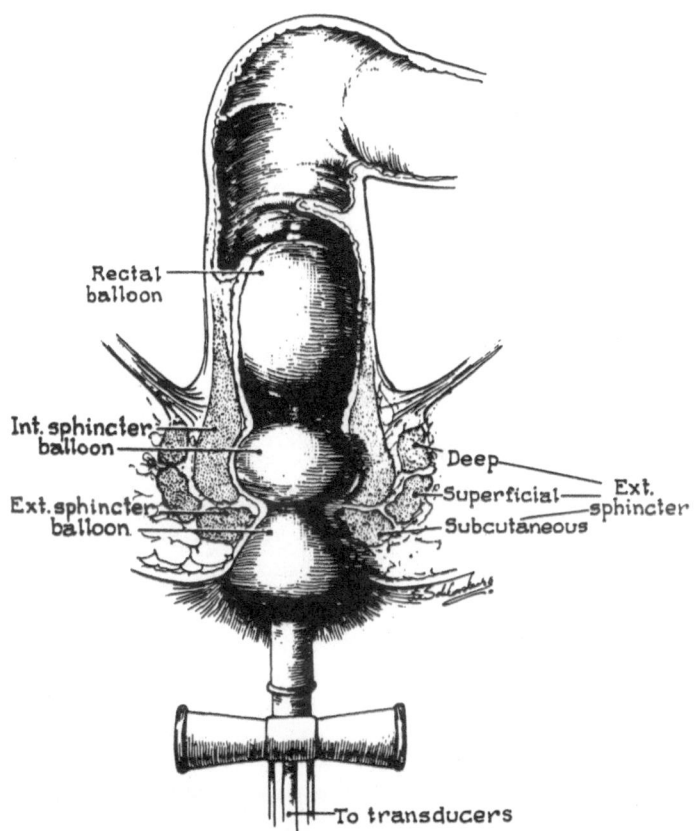

Rectal balloon

Int. sphincter balloon

Ext. sphincter balloon

Deep

Superficial — Ext. sphincter

Subcutaneous

To transducers

Figure 8.8 Schematic diagram of the apparatus for distending the rectum and recording pressure changes within the internal and external anal sphincters (From Schuster *et al.*, 1965, with kind permission of the authors and the editor of Bull. Johns Hopkins Hosp.)

monitored in man by a series of suitably placed balloons (Figure 8.8). Distension of the rectum results in relaxation of the internal anal sphincter and contraction of the external anal sphincter. If distension is brief, the associated relaxation of the internal sphincter is also brief. However, during maintained distension the relaxation adapts so that the contracted state resumes even as the rectum remains distended (Figure 8.9). The act of defaecation can be suppressed by the contraction of the external sphincter and is a major factor in anal continence.

If defaecation is not suppressed a complex sequence of events follows which is coordinated entirely within the sacral cord and mediated by sacral parasympathetic reflexes. Peristaltic action in the sigmoid colon and contraction of the longitudinal muscle in the rectum and distal colon shorten the rectum so that the angle between between them disappears. Pressure rises in the rectum and as the internal and external sphincters relax contents are expelled.

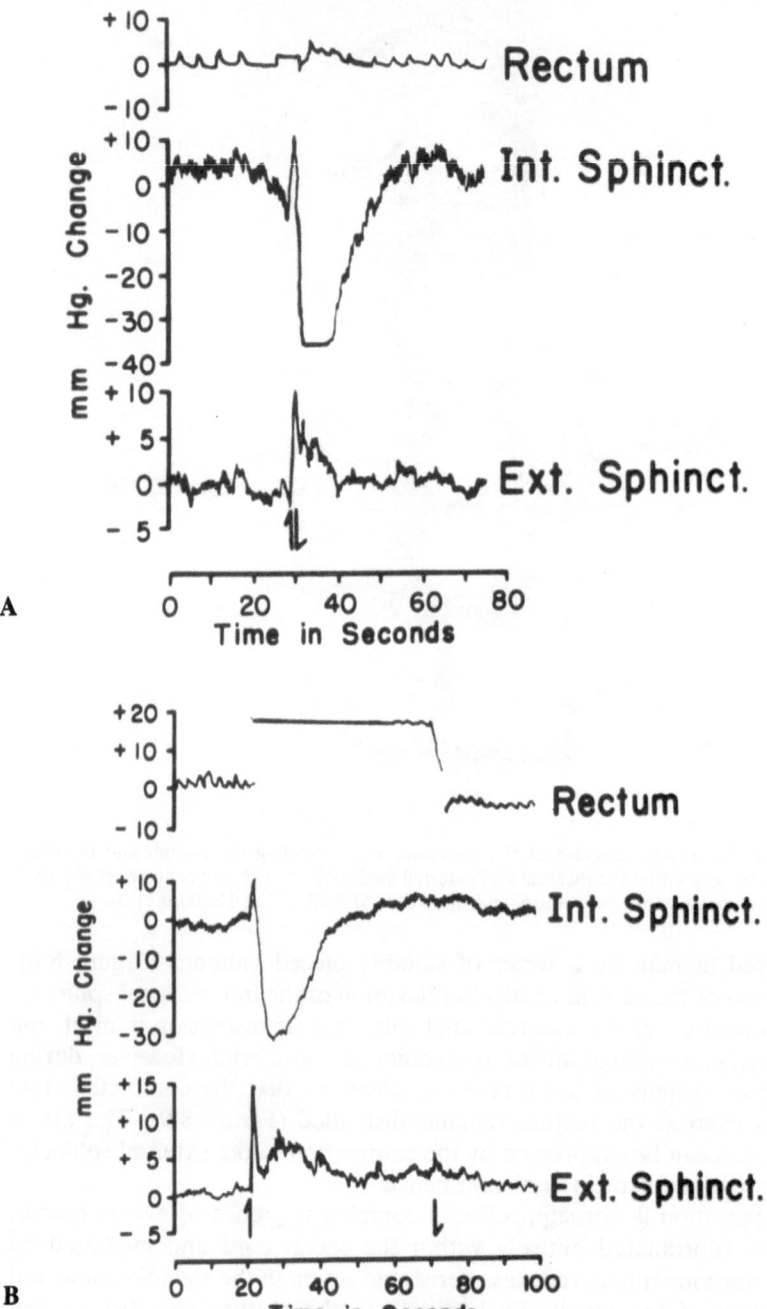

Figure 8.9 Sphincteric responses to brief (**A**) and maintained (**B**) distension of the rectum (arrows) (From Schuster *et al.*, 1965, with kind permission of the authors and the editor of Bull. Johns Hopkins Hosp.)

Evacuation is normally facilitated by central nervous mechanisms which raise the intra-abdominal pressure. Forced expiration against a closed glottis raises both thoracic and abdominal pressure. The haemodynamic consequences of this 'Valsalva's manoeuvre' are quite marked following a reduction in venous return to the heart, and death while straining at stool is not uncommon. Contraction of abdominal muscles also raises abdominal pressure which together with raised intraluminal pressure brought about by powerful propulsive contractions in the descending colon aid evacuation.

The voluntary facilitation and inhibition of defaecation illustrate the involvement of the cerebral cortex. Descending pathways project to the sacral cord and modify local reflexes. When voluntary closure of the external anal sphincter is used to delay the act of defaecation the faeces remain in the rectum which relaxes to accommodate its increased volume. This relaxation, by decreasing tension in the muscle wall, reduces the mechanoreceptive input and removes the stimulus, so the urge to defaecate subsides. Consequently the rectum may still be distended but the defaecation reflex is not activated until subsequent mass movements again increase the rectal volume and raise intraluminal pressure. Water reabsorption continues in the rectum so that a prolonged stay there results in further solidification of faecal matter with subsequent difficulty in expulsion.

9
The coordination of gastrointestinal motility: the fasted state

INTRODUCTION

Transit of a meal through the stomach and small intestine is rapid compared to its long stay in the caecum and colon. In animals which take discrete meals as opposed to *ad libitum* eaters, the meal is almost completly digested within only a few hours of eating; the nutrients released from this process have been absorbed and undigested residues are collecting in the colon. The large intestine is just starting its work as that of the proximal bowel is coming to an end.

Originally, at this stage in the process the stomach and small intestine were thought to enter a state of 'suspended animation' awaiting the arrival of the next meal. The blood supply, secretory processes and motor activity were all believed to shut down during the interdigestive period. However, it is now recognized that these proximal regions are far from quiescent in the fasted state. Instead a pattern of periodic activity involving both secretion and motility develops 4–5 hours after a meal and continues relentlessly until food is again ingested.

The motility present during this fasted state consists of a brief period of intense contractile activity, followed by a long period of inactivity with contractions then developing gradually until an intense burst again appears about 2 hours after the last one. Activity begins in the stomach and duodenum and propagates slowly towards the ileum, a new burst of contractile activity developing proximally each time activity approaches the terminal ileum. There is, therefore, always one region of the stomach or small intestine in a state of intense contractile activity.

Before this interdigestive pattern of motility was recognized, early workers noted the variability of gastric and intestinal motility recorded from conscious animals. On some occasions a particular region of the gut was totally inactive while at other times, under identical circumstances, the gut was extremely active. However, in these early papers most emphasis was placed on the classification of individual contraction waveforms and few recordings were made for the length of time necessary to identify the cyclical motor pattern. Boldyreff (1905) described motor events in the stomach of the fasting dog which approximate closely with present views. Unfortunately, because of Boldyreff's interpretation of the results, the implications of these findings were not recognized and the paper faded into obscurity (see Wingate (1981) for a comprehensive historical account).

Full recognition of the cyclical nature of interdigestive motility came more than 60 years after the publication of Boldyreff's initial findings and was brought about by technical developments in electromyography. This technique allows the electrical events associated with contractions to be recorded, for prolonged periods, simultaneously from serosal electrodes placed at regular intervals along the gastrointestinal tract. It was in this way that motility in fasted animals was confirmed as a cyclical event, but it established, moreover, the interdigestive activity as a migrating phenomenon which propagates along the whole length of small bowel (Szurszewski, 1969). The recurring sequence of electrical events was given the name migrating myoelectrical complex (MMC). However, the strong correlation between myoelectrical and motor events allows the more functional descriptive term of migrating motor complex to adopt the same abbreviation.

THE MIGRATING MOTOR COMPLEX

A systematic study of MMC activity in the stomach and small intestine of the dog was made by Code and Marlett (1975) who defined four characteristic phases of the MMC cycle as it passed over a single recording site (Figure 9.1). Phase I is the quiescent phase when only slow waves can be detected electromyographically. This period lasts between 30 min and an hour, being of generally shorter duration in the stomach, and is followed by a period of similar duration when persistent but random spike activity is superimposed on the slow wave oscillations. This is phase II (also referred to as a period of irregular spiking activity or ISA) where continuous spike activity increases in incidence and intensity until the onset of the phase III. During the latter phase each slow wave has action potentials of maximal duration and amplitude superimposed (hence it is also called the period of regular spiking activity, or RSA). This phase is also referred to as the activity front and lasts for approximately 4–7 min in the small intestine but longer in the stomach. Phase IV is when spiking activity rapidly subsides and merges into phase I. Because phase III of the complex is most easily recognizable, and because it generally starts and finishes abruptly, the total

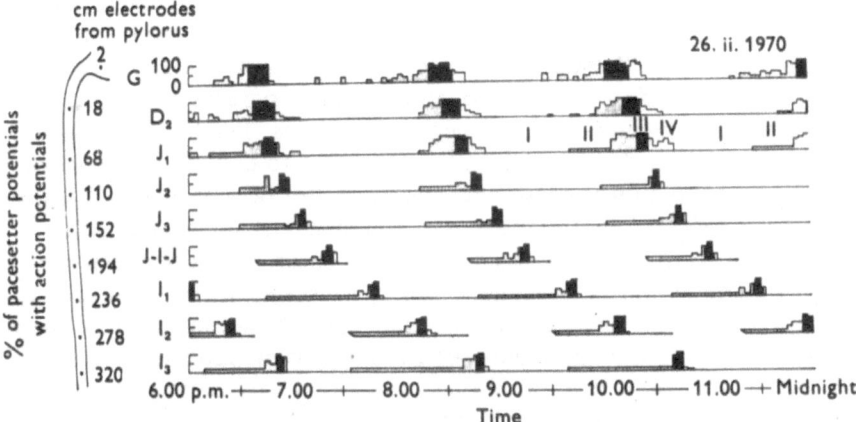

Figure 9.1 Fasting motor activity in the conscious dog recorded myoelectrically and plotted as a percentage of slow waves with superimposed spikes. Three complexes occurred in the 6 h recording session and are seen to migrate from the stomach to the terminal ileum. As one complex ends in the ileum another starts in the stomach and duodenum so that there is always activity present at some point in the small intestine. Four phases of each complex are identified at each recording site with the dark bands representing phase III or the activity fronts (From Code and Marlett, 1975, with kind permission of the authors and the editor of J. Physiol. (London))

duration of a migrating motor complex is usually measured from one phase III to the next. The mean periods of the cycles ranges from 90 to 120 min.

Recording from several sites simultaneously illustrates the aboral progression of the MMC sequence from the stomach to the distal ileum (see Figure 9.1). Phase III activity begins almost simultaneously in the stomach and duodenum and then migrates distally over the entire small bowel. The rate of this migration slows considerably as the MMC propagates distally from 6–12 cm min^{-1} in the stomach and duodenum to between 1 and 2 cm min^{-1} at the terminal ileum. The consequence of this is the length of bowel simultaneously engaged in phase III activity. In the stomach and duodenum 40–60 cm is simultaneously affected whilst in the terminal ileum only between 5 and 10 cm is affected. The segment of bowel distal to that undergoing phase III contractions shows irregular phase II activity while the bowel proximal is inactive.

In the dog the activity front takes between 100 and 130 min to travel from the start in the stomach to the end at the ileocaecal sphincter. This is approximately the same as the total cycle time at a single locus and so it appears that as one MMC reaches the end of the small intestine another begins in the stomach (see Figure 9.1). However, some MMCs (about 20%) start distal to the stomach and not all (again about 20%) reach the terminal ileum.

The motor activity in the human stomach and small intestine shows the same cyclical motor pattern. In a recent study the total duration of the

MMC was reported to be 82 ± 5 min (mean $\pm$ SE in 38 volunteers) with complexes starting mainly in the duodenum. Only about 20% started in the stomach while 9% started distal to the ligament of Treitz. The activity front had a 4.5 min duration and propagated at 6.8 cm s^{-1} in the upper small intestine (Peeters, Vantrappen and Janssens, 1982).

The function of the MMC has been compared to one of a 'houskeeper' which cleans up after the last meal and thereafter periodically sweeps the bowel clear of cell debris and bacteria. In humans lacking phase III activity, bacterial overgrowth of the small intestine is observed (Vantrappen *et al.*, 1977). Another function of the MMC is suggested to be analogous to 'fitness training' so that the stomach and small bowel are kept in good muscular condition by periodic exercise during prolonged fasts.

CONTROL OF THE MIGRATING MOTOR COMPLEX

Since the arrival of an activity front at the terminal ileum generally coincides with the development of a new phase III in the lower oesophageal sphincter and stomach it was originally suggested that these two events were linked, the MMC in the ileum triggering the proximal one (Szurszewski, 1969). However, in man especially, not all MMCs reach the terminal

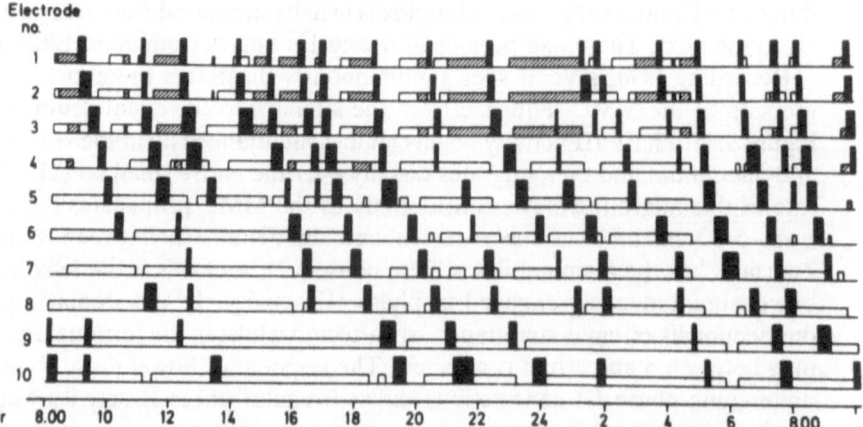

Figure 9.2 Composite diagram of 26 hr continuous recording from 10 electrodes along the entire small intestine of a normal fasting subject. Phase II is the open blocks and phase III the black blocks. The hatched blocks represent the presence of minute rhythms which were only apparent in the jejunal segment during phase II (From Fleckenstein and Oigaard, 1978, with kind permission of the authors and the editor of Dig. Dis. Sci.)

ileum and some start distal to the stomach and duodenum (Figure 9.2). This would indicate that there is no cause and effect relationship between activity in these two regions. This is further emphasized by pharmacological treatments which can initiate 'ectopic' MMCs. Injections of morphine, for example. initiate premature phase III activity in the duodenum of both fed and fasted animals which then propagates distally (Sarna, Northcott and Belbeck, 1982). When premature MMCs are elicited they occur before the previous complex has reached the end of the small intestine, so that several separate complexes can be present simultaneously at different levels of the gastrointestinal tract. The mechanisms responsible for the initiation of MMC activity and those regulating its propagation distally would therefore appear to be independent.

The two main questions, therefore, are:

(1)   What controls the initiation of the MMC and where in the proximal gut it originate?
(2)   What is the mechanism of propagation along the bowel?

Another consideration tied in with the first question relates to the duration of the different phases of MMC activity and the level of contraction present in the individual phases.

Propagation of the migrating motor complex

It is now evident that the enteric nervous system is the medium through which the MMC is propagated. Earlier work, however, suggested that the extrinsic nerves were responsible in much the same way as propagation of peristaltic waves along the oesophagus depend on a craniocaudal sequence of nervous activation. This idea came about from experiments on loops of intestine separated from the main bowel so that the intrinsic innervation was disrupted but their extrinsic supply intact (Thiry–Vella loop); the continuity of the bowel was restored by anastomosing the proximal and distal stumps of bowel. Carlson, Bedi and Code (1972) using this preparation found that the majority of complexes showed a normal progression along the small intestine. Thus complexes migrated to the point of anastomosis, jumped across to and along the Thiry–Vella loop and then back to the bowel distal to the anastomosis and on towards the end of the small intestine. The only way this could happen is if the extrinsic nerves were coordinating the progress of the MMC.

Evidence against such a role for the extrinsic nerves is indicated in other experiments where the continuity of the intramural nerves is prevented by either bowel transection or pharmacological intervention. In the study by Bueno, Praddaude and Ruckebusch (1979) the normal progression through a Thiry–Vella loop was seen only for a few MMCs while the majority failed to enter the loop or did so only after a significant delay. Other complexes appeared de novo in the loop. They suggested that the MMCs do not propagate beyond the anastomosis but that new complexes are organized in the loop.

Transecting the bowel and then reanastomosed in its original site also stops the propagation of the MMC (Figure 9.3). A series of such sections

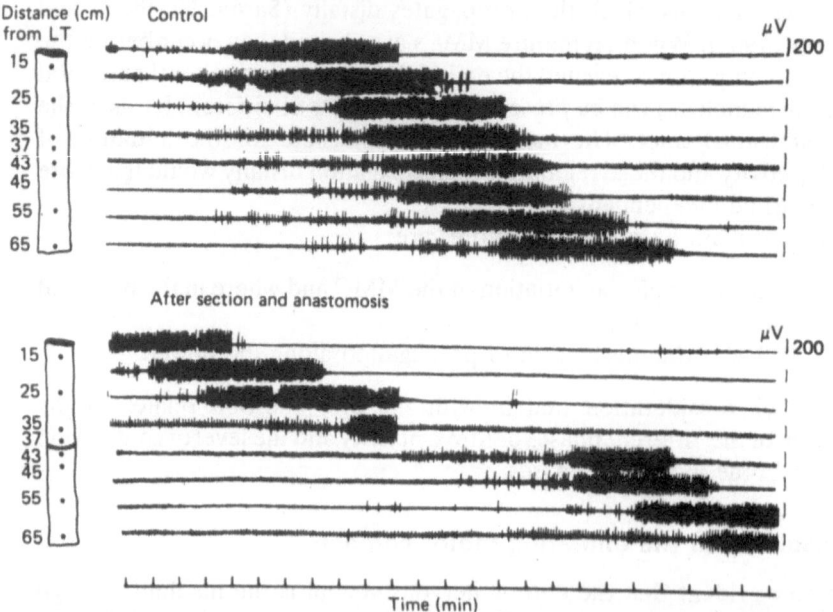

Figure 9.3 Electrical activity recorded from the conscious dog showing the propagation of phase III activity along the jejunum from 15 to 65 cm beyond the ligament of Treitz (LT). Position of the electrodes is shown diagramatically on the left. After transection and reanastomosis of the jejunum at the point indicated propagation appears to be delayed for 10 min at the site of anastomosis. However, the complex below the section was probably unrelated to that above (From Bueno, Praddaude and Ruckebusch, 1979, with kind permission of the authors and the editor of J. Physiol. (London))

results in loops of bowel that all generate MMC activity independent from that in the adjacent segments, and furthermore has a different MMC period (Sarna, Condon and Cowles, 1983) (Figure 9.4). Some complexes appear to have bridged the gap created by the transection. However, when the time-lag between MMCs in adjacent segments is analysed and compared to that seen before transection it becomes apparent that these are chance occurences caused by the variable and random temporal relationship between MMCs in the two segments. The arrival of one MMC at the end of one segment and the start of another in the next segment are two independent complexes.

The injection of low doses of pharmacological blocking agents into the artery supplying a particular loop of intestine has effects only on that loop since dilution of the drug as it passes into the venous effluent and on through the systemic circulation reduces the concentration to subthreshold levels. Atropine, hexamethonium, or tetrodotoxin, injected close arterially, stop the distal propagation of MMCs (Sarna *et al.*, 1981a). The proximal-to-distal propagation would appear, therefore, to be mediated through intrinsic cholinergic nerves.

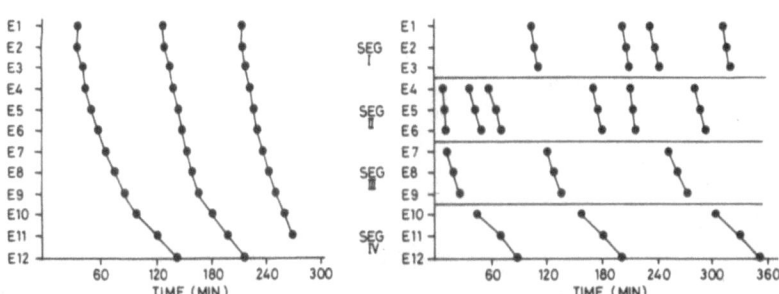

Figure 9.4 Propagation of MMC activity along the small intestine of the dog before (left) and after (right) transection and reanastamosis of the bowel to make four segments of intestine. The dots indicate the end of phase III and the lines indicate their propagation. (Reprinted by permission of Elsevier Science Publishing Co. Inc., from: Enteric mechanisms of initiation of migrating myoelectric complexes in dogs, by Sarna, S., Condon, R. E. and Cowles, V. *Gastroenterology*, **84**, 814–22. Copyright 1983 by The American Gastroenterological Association.)

These experiments would therefore exclude the extrinsic nervous system as the means of propagation. Further support for this conclusion can be drawn from experiments in which *in situ* regions of small intestine are extrinsically denervated with only minor modification in the distal propagation of MMC (Figure 9.5). However, the frequency of these complexes and their rate of propagation are altered by extrinsic denervation, suggesting that reflexes within the extrinsic nerves may affect the periodicity and propagation of the MMC (Bueno *et al.*, 1979; Hepple, Kelly and Sarr, 1983).

The initiation of the migrating motor complex

Two main hypotheses have been proposed for the initiation of the MMC: hormonal and neural.

MMCs can start at various locations; in some instances they can originate as high as the lower oesophageal sphincter and stomach, while at other times they appear to start much lower in the duodenum or jejunum. MMCs are therefore not organized at a unique site. They occur in the stomach after removal of a large part of the distal small intestine and arise in the duodenum after removal of the stomach. Thus neither the stomach or intestine are essential for the initiation of complexes. However, communication between them via the enteric nervous system allows proximal-to-distal propagation. Thus after transection and reanastomosis of the small intestine each segment is capable of initiating MMC activity but because communication between segments is lost the complexes occur independently. The intrinsic nervous system is therefore important for the initiation of complexes as well as for their aboral propagation.

Any site can generate MMCs but when the bowel is intact they usually arise at a proximal site and propagate aborally to the terminal ileum. The

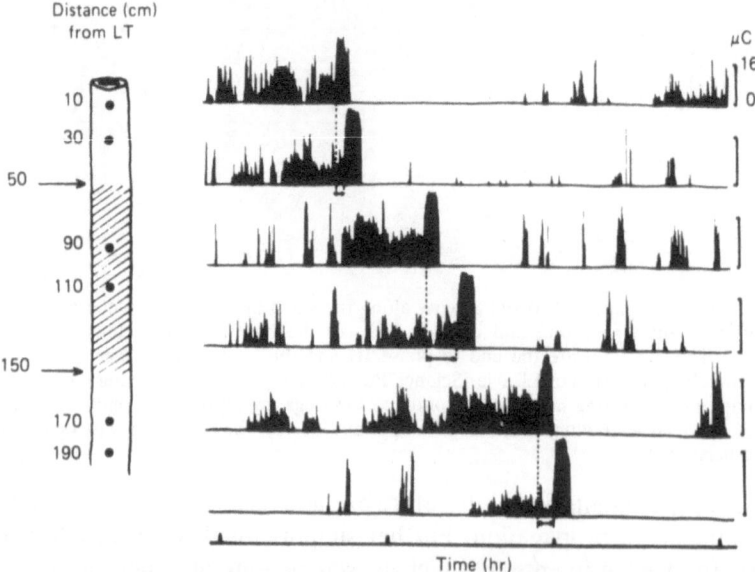

Figure 9.5 Electrical spiking activity of the jejunum integrated at 20 s intervals showing propagation of an MMC through a 1 m segment of jejunum denervated by section of the mesenteric nerves (hatched region). The velocity of propagation is indicated from the interval between the onset of phase III activity at the pairs of recording electrodes. The propagation velocity is less in the denervated segment (From Bueno, Praddaude and Ruckebusch, 1979, with kind permission of the authors and the editor of J. Physiol. (London))

initiation and normal progression, under these circumstances, is largely independent of the extrinsic nerves although, as will be seen later, the vagus may influence proximal regions. Thus, chronic vagotomy, removal of the coeliac and superior mesenteric ganglia, or division of the paravascular nerves surrounding the superior mesenteric artery does not prevent the initiation of the MMC, although each may affect the timing of the complex.

A hormonal mediator is therefore a distinct possibility and such a mechanism was indicated in the dog by the continued cyclical activity in a gastric pouch autotransplanted into the pelvic region (Thomas and Kelly, 1979). Such a procedure ensures that all intrinsic and extrinsic nervous connections are permanently severed yet the cyclical activity in the pouch coincided with that in the remaining stomach and duodenum.

Since the MMC is cyclical and propagates the length of the stomach and small intestine, each phase of the complex is always present at some point. Any hormone involved in the initiation process must therefore have a plasma concentration which cycles in phase with the MMCs in the most proximal region. The gastrointestinal hormones which show such a relationship are shown in Figure 9.6. However, the question arises: do the changes in hormone level mediate the MMC or are they a consequence of the cycles in motor activity?

THE FASTED STATE

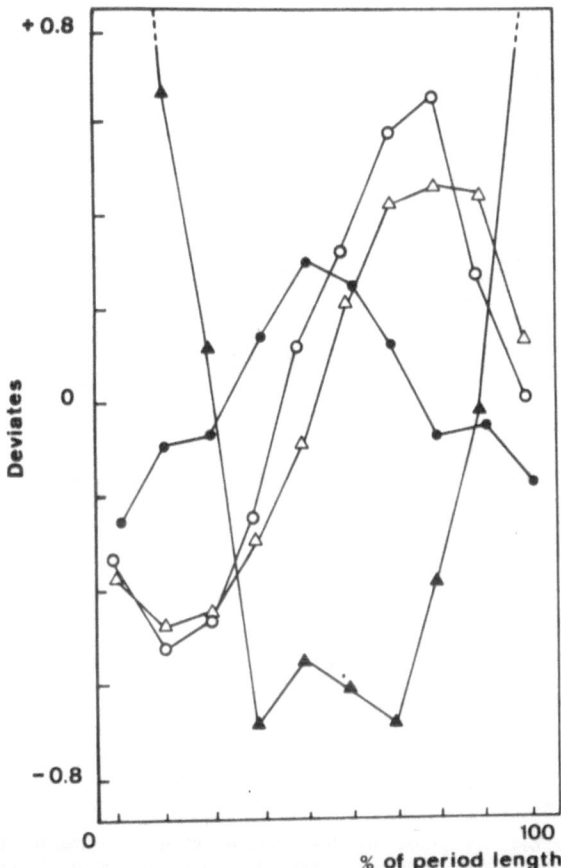

Figure 9.6 Relationship between endogenous fluctuations of gastrin (filled circles), motilin (open triangles), pancreatic polypeptide (open circles) and somatostatin (filled triangles), and the migrating motor complex. The start of an activity front in the upper duodenum is taken as a reference point to delineate periods. The ordinate represents mean standard deviates (From Peeters, Vantrappen and Janssens, 1982, with kind permission of the authors and publisher, F.K. Schattauer Verlag)

Motilin, a 22 aminoacid residue polypeptide isolated from the porcine duodenum (Brown, Cook and Dryburgh, 1973), is the strongest contender for the hormonal mediator since the intravenous infusion of this peptide in both dog and man induces premature complexes that are similar in appearance and migration to the naturally occurring ones (Figure 9.7). The larger the dose of motilin the sooner a second complex is initiated, while the longer the delay after the preceding complex the less the amount of motilin that has to be infused. The sensitivity to motilin therefore alters during the MMC cycle such that there is a relative refractory period immediately after the passage of one activity front which diminishes during the following phase I.

GASTROINTESTINAL MOTILITY

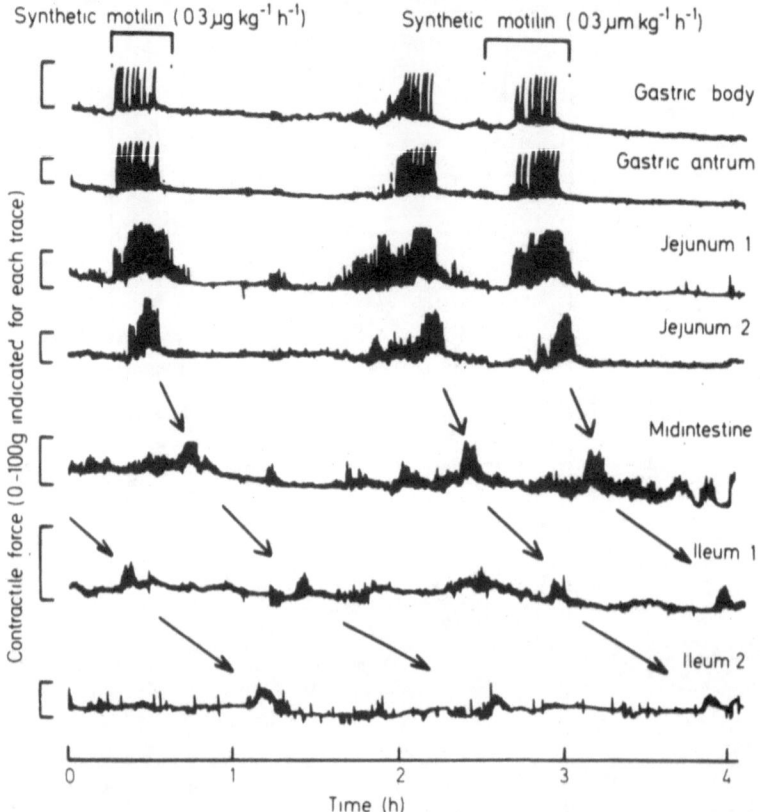

Figure 9.7 Effect of i.v. infusion of motilin on gastrointestinal contractile activity in a fasted dog (Reprinted from: Motilin-induced mechanical activity in the canine alimentary tract, by Itoh, Z. and Sekiguchi, T. from the Scandinavian Journal of Gastroenterology, by permission of Universitetsforlaget, Oslo.)

Endogenous plasma motilin levels show a peak at about the same time that phase III activity develops in the stomach, and is lowest during phase I (Figure 9.8). Endogenous motilin levels have therefore been postulated to initiate the MMC. However, this hypothesis is not flawless. On some occasions phase III activity occurs without a corresponding increase in plasma motilin, and at other times peaks in motilin occur without an activity front. Other procedures can also influence the relationship between motilin and the MMC. For example, antisera raised against motilin will reduce the background motilin level for several days but have only a transient effect on MMC activity (Konturek, 1984). Thus the association between motilin and the MMC is not clear cut.

Sarna *et al.* (1984), after looking closely at the relationship between MMC activity and plasma motilin levels concluded that peaks in motilin concentration occurred several minutes after the onset of phase III in the

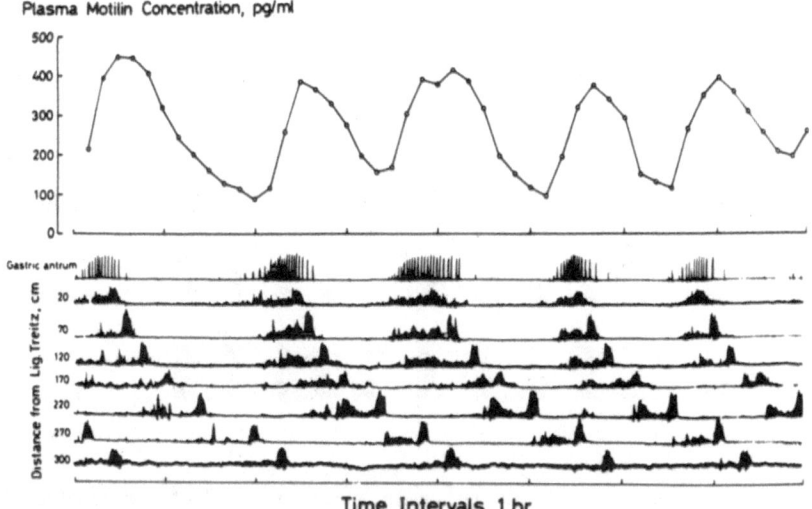

Figure 9.8 Close relationship between the plasma motilin concentration and occurrence of MMC activity in the dog (Reprinted from: Interdigestive motor activity in health and disease, by Itoh, Z. and Sekiguchi, T. from the Scandinavian Journal of Gastroenterology, by permission of Universitetsforlaget, Oslo.)

duodenum and suggested that in this 'chicken and egg controversy the MMC wins'. In other words, the motilin peaks as a consequence of the complex and not vice versa. However, the peak itself may not necessarily be the trigger, as a 'critical' level of motilin may occur before the peak, or the rate of rise in motilin concentration may be more important than absolute levels. The MMC–motilin controversy is yet to be resolved.

Other hormones also initiate premature complexes. Substance P, somatostatin and neurotensin, when infused into fasted dogs, increase the occurrence rate of the MMC (Konturek, 1984). Endogenous somatostatin levels oscillate with the MMC cycle, but when infused in man inhibit all gastric MMC activity yet evoke phase III activity in the intestine at intervals considerably less than the normal cycle (Figure 9.9).

Of the other hormones that show oscillation in their endogenous plasma level, pancreatic polypeptide and gastrin do not affect the initiation of MMCs at physiological doses. However, preliminary evidence suggests that pancreatic polypeptide inhibits the gastric phase III component while gastrin stimulates phase II activity (Peeters *et al.*, 1982). These hormones would therefore appear to be modulators, rather than initiators, of MMC activity. Interactions between different hormones, and between nerves and hormones, may prove to be important in determining the overall levels of motility in different regions of the gastrointestinal tract during both the fed and fasted state.

Although the precise role of these and possibly other hormones in the overall control is not fully known, what is clear from the description above

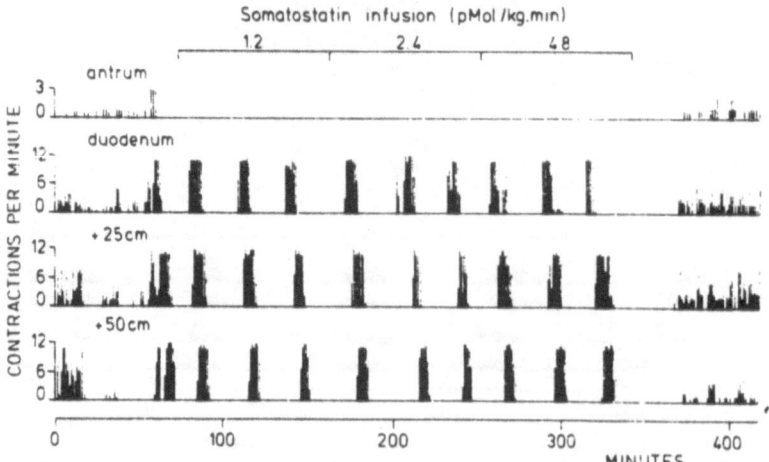

Figure 9.9 Representation of the manometric recording from the human small intestine during a control period and three consecutive periods of somatostatin infusion (From Peeters, Janssen and Vantrappen, 1983, with kind permission of the authors and the editor of Regulatory Peptides)

is that the gastric and intestinal MMC can be influenced independently. This is further emphasized by the different degree of dependence on vagal integrity as shown recently by the technique of vagal cooling. In these experiments dogs were prepared with their cervical vagi isolated in loops of skin. Cooling thermodes could then be placed around the vagi enabling conduction in the nerves to be rapidly and reversibly blocked in the conscious animal merely by reducing the temperature in the nerves to below 4 °C. With the nerves at body temperature the normal progression of MMC activity from the lower oesophageal sphincter and stomach through the duodenum and jejunum was established. Upon cooling the vagi all cyclical activity in the lower oesophageal sphincter and stomach disappeared. In the intestine MMC activity continued with the same period-icity but without any phase II activity preceding the activity fronts (Figure 9.10).

These results suggesting considerable vagal influence on MMC activity are quite different from previous studies in which the nerves are sectioned during a surgical operation. Since the effect of the nerve section can only be investigated some time later it is possible that the differences are due to some reinnervation by the vagus nerves, or possibly adaptation of the enteric nervous system to the lack of a vagal innervation. The conclusions from the vagal cooling experiments might be that these nerves regulate MMCs in the lower oesophageal sphincter and stomach but not in the intestine. During vagal cooling the cycles in pancreatic polypeptide and gastrin levels in the blood were also abolished but motilin levels continued to oscillate with the intestinal complex even though no gastric activity was

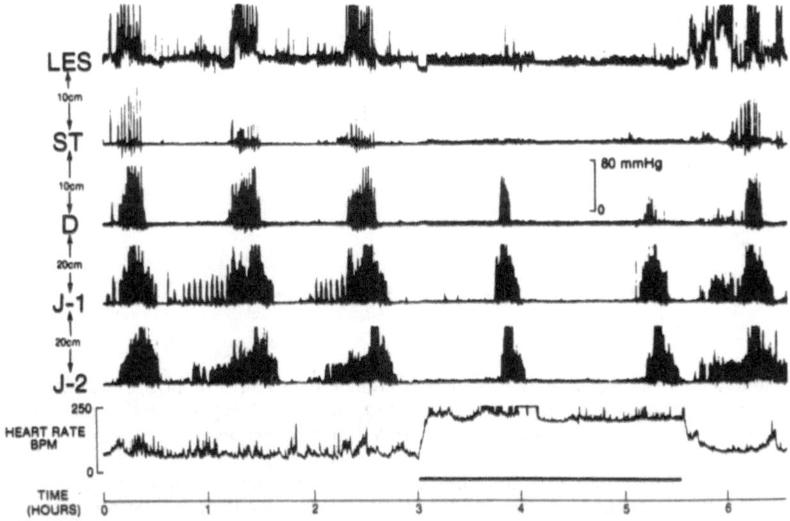

Figure 9.10 The effect of bilateral vagal blockade on canine MMC activity recorded manometrically. Period of vagal blockade is marked by bar and its effectiveness indicated by the increase in heart rate. Recording sites indicated on left are lower (o)esophageal sphincter (LES), stomach (ST), duodenum (D) and jejunum (J) (From Hall, El-Sharkawy and Diamant, 1982, with kind permission of the authors and the editor of Am. J. Physiol.)

present (Hall *et al.*, 1983). Motilin is therefore unlikely to be solely responsible for initiating gastric MMC activity but could trigger the duodenal MMC.

How might vagal activity control MMC activity in the lower oesophageal sphincter and stomach? One possibility would be that a 'clock' in the central nervous system produces a vagal discharge which increases during phase II up to a maximum during phase III and which stimulates the smooth muscle in the lower oesophageal sphincter and stomach to contract. The efferent discharge recorded from the reinnervated diaphragm of the fasted dog does indeed show such a pattern (Figure 9.11). However, because the efferent fibres are reflexly modulated by afferent inputs from the stomach and intestine, it is equally possible that the motor activity associated with the different phases of the MMC reflexly drives the efferent discharge, and not the other way round.

An alternative way of achieving the same end result would be for a constant unmodulated efferent discharge to provide a background of vagal tone which allows the expression of MMC activity but does not necessarily drive it. In this situation the initiation and timing of the complex would depend on an alternative peripheral mechanism. Such an alternative may be a 'clock' within the enteric nervous system which resets each time an activity front has developed. As the clock 'ticks' towards the next phase III the level of motility gradually increases from zero in phase I, through

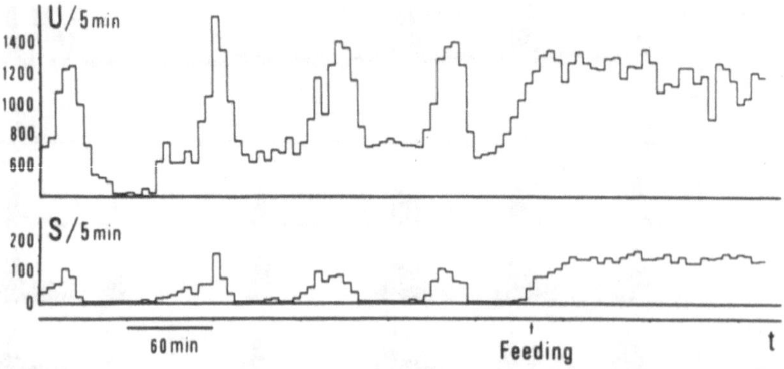

Figure 9.11 Discharge pattern of a vagal efferent fibre probably supplying the antrum during fasting and feeding in conscious dog. U/5 min, number of vagal impulses per 5 min as a function of time; recording made using a nerve suture technique; S/5 min, number of gastric spike potentials per 5 min as a function of time; recording made with electrodes chronically implanted in the antrum wall. In fasting dog, there are cyclical variations of vagal discharge with parallel variations in gastric motility (MMCs). Feeding increases both vagal discharge and gastric motility (From Miolan and Roman, 1978b, with kind permission of the authors and the editor of Am. J. Physiol.)

a phase of intermediate activity until finally there is the maximum activity of phase III. The 'clock' may be advanced or retarded by external influences such as the vagus nerve or circulating hormones. In addition, the expression of the 'clock' in terms of the level of motility and duration of the different phases may also be subject to external modifications. External influences therefore act not as triggering agents but modulators of the local enteric mechanisms. The output from the 'clock' is via the intramural cholinergic innervation of the muscle layers. Anything affecting the level of activity in this cholinergic pathway may also modify the MMC. Finally, substances may act directly on the muscle itself. These substances would therefore alter the contractile state of the bowel without affecting the 'clock' itself.

Sarna *et al.* (1983) suggested an enteric mechanism for the initiation of the MMC on the basis of their transection experiments. After the small bowel had been transected and reanastomosed into four segments whose intrinsic nervous connections were severed, each segment generated independent MMCs which propagated over the length of the segment but not into adjacent regions. The time period of the MMCs were, with the exception of the most proximal segment, progressively longer in more distal segments. Between 60 and 100 days after the transections normal progression of complexes returned presumably because of nerve regeneration within the intrinsic plexus.

The analogy between the proximal-to-distal gradient in slow wave frequency and a similar gradient in frequency of MMC cycles led the authors to propose that a series of MMC relaxation oscillators, each with its own intrinsic frequency, were present throughout the gut. They proposed that

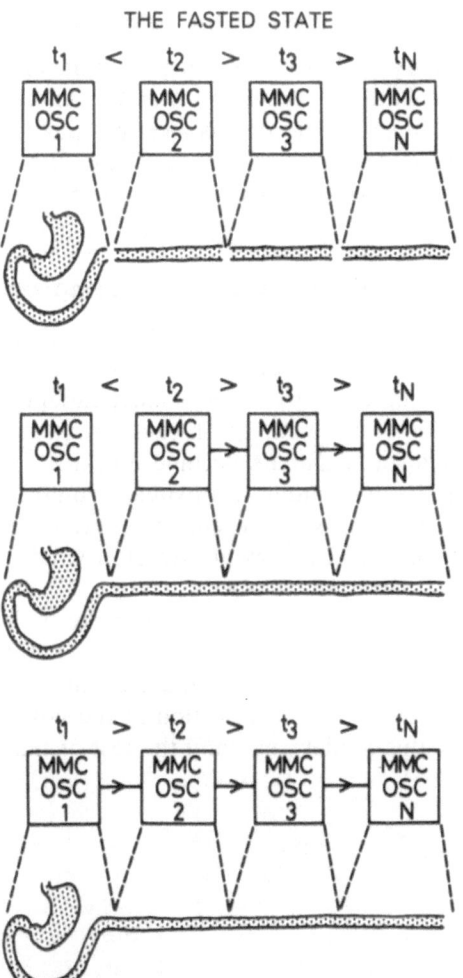

Figure 9.12 Diagram showing proposed model of MMC oscillators. Top panel: Each segment of the small intestine behaves like an independent MMC relaxation oscillator. When segments of bowel are isolated from each other by transection and reanastomosis, each segment has its own periodicity (represented by t) with the second region (MMC OSC 2) having the highest frequency (indicated by <> signs). When coupled through the intrinsic nerve plexuses, this region acts as pacemaker for more distal segments so that MMC originate in this region and propagate towards the distal ileum (middle panel). In the lower panel the most proximal region is dominant so that MMCs propagate the full length of the bowel (Modified from Sarna *et al.*, 1983, and Wingate, 1983)

coupling between these oscillators would provide entrainment such that the oscillator with the highest frequency would dominate and generate the normal progression seen *in situ*. The segment with the highest frequency is not the most proximal one but that corresponding to the jejunal region. This may account for the number of MMCs that originate in this region and not the stomach and duodenum (see Figure 9.2). MMCs, however, frequently originate in the lower oesophageal sphincter and stomach and propagate the full length of the small intestine. An explanation for this may be related to the sensitivity of this most proximal region to its vagal supply and to endogenous hormone levels. These factors may be able to decrease the interval between MMC cycles and thus allow this region to dominate.

Model for the control of migrating motor complexes

Figure 9.12 shows the proposed model of MMC oscillators. In this model four such oscillators are shown, each with its individual intrinsic frequency. When these are uncoupled, MMCs occur independently at each site, but when coupled the oscillator with the highest frequency (no. 2) acts as pacemaker so that distal segments become entrained. When this occurs MMCs originate in the duodenum or proximal jejunum. However, should the period of the most proximal oscillator shorten so that this region became the pacemaker a MMC would develop which would sweep the entire tract.

This model fits the available data relating to the variable site of origin of the MMC, the different sensitivities of proximal and distal regions to vagal blockade and various hormones, and accounts for the ability of any region to generate MMCs after transection of the bowel wall. It remains to be seen whether this model can stand the test of time.

10
The coordination of gastrointestinal motility: the fed state

INTRODUCTION

Feeding, in animals which eat discrete meals, results in the interruption of the periodic migrating motor complex described in Chapter 9. It is replaced by contractile activity which is present simultaneously throughout the

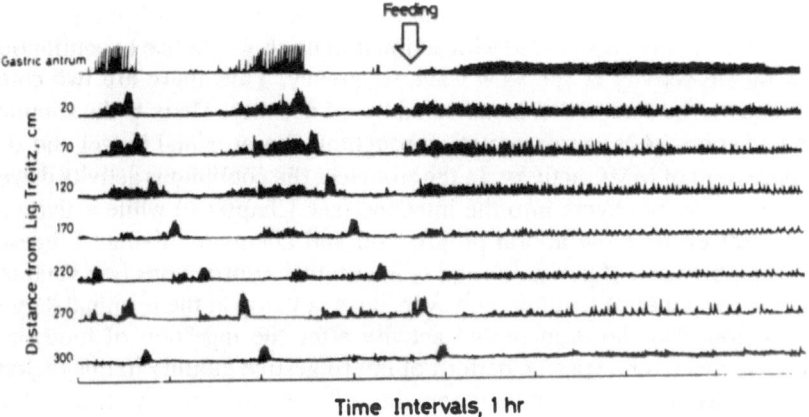

Figure 10.1 Eight hour recording of contractile activity in the gastrointestinal tract of a conscious dog. Note the continuous pattern of motility after feeding (Reprinted from Interdigestive motor activity in health and disease by Itoh, Z. and Sekiguchi, T. from the Scandinavian Journal of Gastroenterology, by permission of Universitetsforlaget, Oslo.)

stomach and small intestine (Figure 10.1), even though the ingested food may have not passed through the pylorus. The changeover, from MMC activity to continuous postprandial activity, occurs almost immediately after the ingestion of food and is maintained for 4–5 hours in man and for much longer in the dog.

In herbivorous animals which feed almost perpetually, the MMC continues uninterrupted, despite the intake of food, so that intestinal contents are moved in batches along the length of intestine ahead of each activity front as it propagates distally. The pig fed *ad libitum*, so that several small meals are taken during the day, shows a similar batch movement of digesta. However, in pigs fed only one or two large meals a day, the MMC is inhibited for between 3 and 6 hours and replaced by the continuous fed type of motor activity (Ruckebusch and Bueno, 1976).

MMC activity would therefore represent a basic motor pattern which is suppressed only in animals, man included, that take large, easily digestible meals. The continuous postprandial motor activity associated with this suppression would ensure the distribution of the highly nutritive digesta over a large area of intestine to allow digestion and subsequent absorption to be optimized.

The postprandial pattern of motility does not have the distinguishing features of the MMC. There are no prolonged periods either of inactivity or of intense contractile activity. Instead the stomach and small intestine show a continuous low level of activity which in many ways resembles the irregular activity seen during phase II of the MMC (see Figure 10.1). However, unlike phase II, it continues for many hours without interruption and when manometric or myoelectrical recordings are compared, the postprandial pattern is less irregular; that is, there is a higher incidence of contractions with much more regular amplitudes. In the antrum especially, all slow waves are associated with action potentials giving rise to continuous contractile activity at the slow wave frequency. Thus there are two components to the conversion from fasted to fed motility. There is the stimulation of continuous motor activity throughout the proximal bowel and the suppression of MMC activity. In the stomach, the continuous activity drives the emptying of chyme into the intestine (see Chapter 6) while activity in the latter ensures the aboral progression and adequate mixing of digesta by a combination of peristaltic and segmentatory contractions (see Chapter 7). The response to feeding, however, does not stop at the terminal ileum. The colon also shows increased activity after the ingestion of food, but because there is no specific pattern of interdigestive motility in this region, and because intestinal contents remain in this region for days rather than hours, the change from the fasted to the fed state is less striking (see Chapter 8).

EFFECT OF MEAL COMPOSITION

The period of interruption of MMC activity and the level of fed-type motility that replaces it depends on the size and the composition of the meal.

The MMC is disrupted more by solid meals than liquid ones. In the dog,

400 ml of milk caused an interruption in MMC activity for approximately 3–4 hours (Code and Marlett, 1975) while a similar-sized meal of meat can delay the reappearance of MMC activity for up to 18 hours. With a particular type of food there is a linear relationship between the amount of food ingested and the period of interrupted MMC. A similar relationship is seen when nutrients are infused directly into the duodenum indicating that the relationship is not due to prolonged gastric emptying. The calorific content of the meal is important. Mixed meals of progressively higher calorific content cause a longer duration of fed motor pattern. However, not all nutrients have the same effect. When equicalorific meals of fat, protein and carbohydrate are compared, fat causes the longest, and protein the shortest, duration of fed response (see Weisbrodt, 1981).

The actual level of postprandial motility, in terms of number of contractions per unit time and overall amplitude of contractions, is also sensitive to meal composition. With equicalorific meals, lipids result in the lowest intensity of postprandial motility (for the greatest duration), proteins the next lowest, while carbohydrate meals generate the highest level of activity. However, even these postprandial contractions are considerably less in amplitude than those encountered during phase III of the MMC.

Thus the level of postprandial motility is adjusted to control the entry of nutrients into the intestine and their subsequent distribution along the length of the small intestine. However, most absorption takes place in the proximal third to one half of the small intestine. Should nutrients appear in the ileum then further adjustments in motility are brought about to slow the rate of gastric emptying and reduce the rate of intestinal transit.

The volume of chyme, its chemical composition and its calorific density are, therefore, all involved in determining the duration of postprandial disruption in the MMC. All these factors alter as the process of digestion and absorption proceed, and so too does the extent of the restraint. Thus, as digestion comes to an end, MMC activity returns again and continues until the next meal.

CONTROL OF POSTPRANDIAL MOTOR ACTIVITY

The changes in motor activity brought about by feeding do not depend on local contact of nutrients with the gastrointestinal mucosa or with the entry of digestion products into the circulation. The latter was discounted by maintaining dogs on total parenteral nutrition for 12 weeks. During this time the animals received nothing by mouth except water and showed no sign of any fed motor pattern (Weisbrodt et al., 1976). The effect of luminal contact with digesta has been investigated in dogs with Thiry–Vella intestinal loops and isolated gastric pouches. Feeding abolished the MMC activity in the isolated segments even though no food came into contact with their mucosal lining. However, perfusion of loops with nutrient fluids did have a direct effect on the motor activity of that segment. Thus as Costa and Furness (1982) point out: 'There seem to be two phases to the initiation of the post-prandial pattern: an early increase in motility which occurs almost simultaneously throughout the small intestine and a delayed, maintained phase of increased motor activity which appears to be related to the arrival of food in the intestine'.

The ingestion of food alters the volume and composition of intraluminal contents which in turn stimulates a variety of reflexes (see Chapter 3) and releases a number of hormones (see Chapter 4). This initiates and maintains the postprandial motor activity. The removal of these stimuli during the course of digestion results in the resumption of the fasting activity. It has been proposed that the various control factors come into action in a sequential manner depending on where in the gastrointestinal tract the stimuli act. As such the situation is analogous to the classification used to describe secretory mechanisms with cephalic, gastric and intestinal phases.

Cephalic phase

By definition, the cephalic phase refers to an increase in motor activity as a consequence of the ingestion of palatable meals such that stimuli arise from outside the gastrointestinal tract usually from visual, olfactory and gustatory sources. The technique used to investigate such effects is 'sham feeding', whereby eating is undertaken but no food enters the stomach. In man this is achieved by spitting out the chewed food, an act which by itself may somewhat lessen the pleasurable aspect of eating, yet it has been reported to disrupt the MMC in the stomach and proximal intestine (Defilippi and Valenzuela, 1981). In animals, such experiments can be more closely controlled by surgical transection of the oesophagus. The cervical oesophagus is divided and the two ends brought separately to the surface and sutured in place. After recovery, the animal is maintained by introducing food either directly into the stomach or into the distal oesophageal opening. However, when the animal is fed 'normally', the food passes out of the proximal opening so that none enters the stomach. Under these conditions in the dog, feeding increased motility in a Thiry–Vella intestinal loop (Gregory, 1950). However, the response persisted only while the act of eating was taking place and declined rapidly once the sham feeding came to an end. Ruckebusch and Bueno (1977) also concluded that the stimulation of intestinal motility by sham feeding was only transient and failed to interrupt the MMC. However, in their experiments sham feeding was achieved by draining the food from a gastric fistula so that although food did reach the stomach the majority of it did not actually remain there.

The effects of sham feeding on secretory processes are mediated via the vagal nerves. Similar beliefs are held for the motor responses but the necessary experiments have yet to be performed. However, cephalic influences mediated pharmacologically by cytoglucopenia have been shown to be mediated via the vagus. This approach involves the systemic injection of insulin or 2-deoxyglucose which reduces the availability of glucose to the hypothalamic 'glucoreceptors' and causes an increase in vagal activity. Such treatments disrupt the MMC and stimulate postprandial motor patterns. Since insulin is released into the circulation during the course of a meal to 'mop up' the nutrients absorbed from the intestine it has been proposed that this may be one mechanism of stimulating postprandial motility. However, after a meal the concentration of insulin in the blood is less than that required to elicit cytoglucopenia, and is also associated with an increase in available glucose, so that hypothalamic stimulation may not arise.

Thus cephalic influences, mediated through the vagus nerves, can stimulate gastric and intestinal motility patterns resembling those seen postprandially. However, these effects are generally shortlived and fail to disrupt the MMC.

Gastric phase

Only when food enters the stomach is there a disruption of the MMC in addition to a stimulation of postprandial activity. Distension of the stomach with an inert stimulus (for example, a balloon) is sufficient to bring about

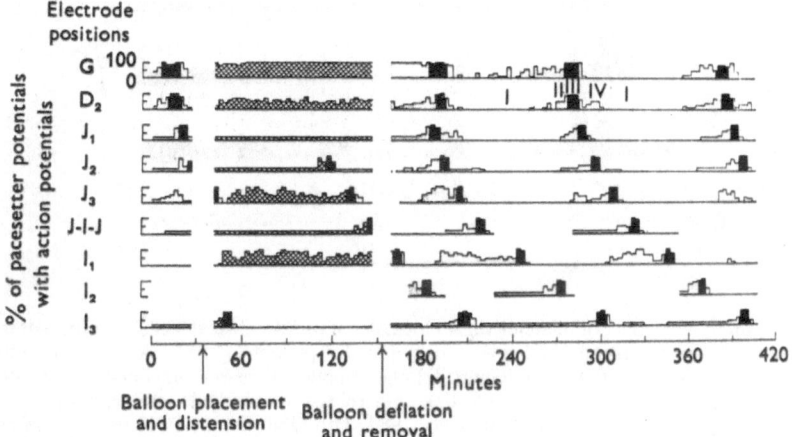

Figure 10.2 Interruption of fasting motor activity in the dog by the inflation of a balloon in the stomach with 400 ml of air (From Code and Marlett, 1975, with kind permission of the authors and the editor of J. Physiol. (London))

these changes but only in proximal regions (Figure 10.2). The distal intestine is relatively insensitive to gastric distension and there is evidence that postprandial activity in proximal and distal regions, like that for the MMC, is controlled differently. The response to gastric distension in the dog is not associated with changes in hormone levels (gastrin, pancreatic polypeptide and motilin) but is abolished by vagotomy. The arrival of food in the stomach is therefore detected by the tension receptors in this region (see Chapter 3) and triggers vagal reflexes which initiate postprandial motor activity.

The importance of these vagal reflexes in the response to food is indicated in the experiments of Diamant *et al.* (1980), in which the vagus nerves in the neck were cooled to prevent the conduction of impulses. Dogs were fed a liquid, meat-based meal which was introduced directly into the stomach via an orogastric tube. This generally resulted in between 7 and 8 hours of postprandial activity. However, cooling the nerves markedly changed the postprandial response. All activity in the stomach was abolished while postprandial activity in the duodenum and jejunum was replaced by MMC activity but modified by the absence of phase II activity

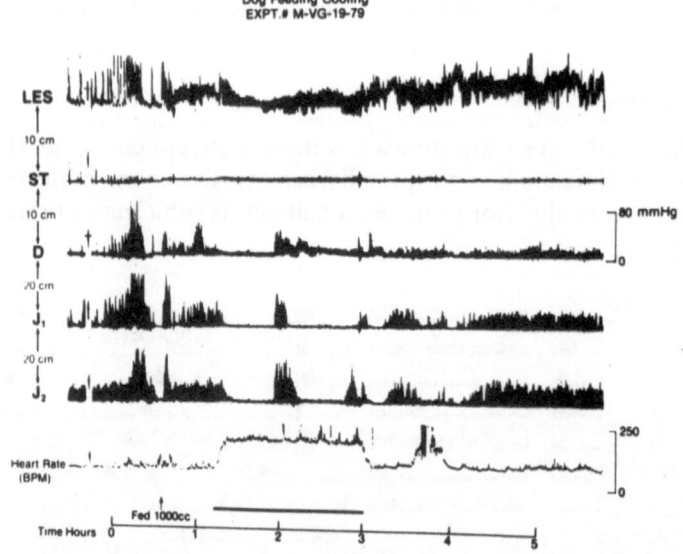

Figure 10.3 The effect of bilateral vagal blockade on the established feeding motor pattern. On nerve blockade (solid bar), lower (o)esophageal pressure (LES) falls, feeding motor activity in the stomach (ST), duodenum (D) and jejunum (J) ceases, and bursts of complex-like activity appear in the small intestine. On release of blockade, the feeding pattern immediately returns (From Diamant *et al.*, 1980, with kind permission of the authors and publisher, Raven Press)

(Figure 10.3) (see also p. 156). Vagal cooling, therefore, resulted in a change from a fed pattern to one typical of the fasted state. On rewarming the nerves the postprandial motility returned.

These experiments indicate a major role for the vagus in the motor response to a meal and in this respect the discharge in vagal efferent fibres increases when food is ingested (see Figure 9.11). Alternatively, the effect of vagal cooling on intestinal motor activity could be explained on the basis of the interruption of gastric emptying that is likely to occur when conduction in the vagus nerves is prevented. However, the abolition of postprandial motility is almost immediate even when cooling is performed after significant quantities of chyme have entered the intestine.

Hormones are also implicated in the gastric phase. Thomas and Kelly (1979) found that motility in an autotransplanted gastric pouch changed from a fasting to a fed pattern after eating. Gastrin has been proposed as a possible hormonal mediator since it is released from the gastric antrum during the course of a meal by both local and reflex mechanisms. Pentagastrin infused into dogs disrupts the MMC and stimulates postprandial-like motility but only in proximal regions. However, gastrin levels return to basal levels after a meal before the return to MMC activity, and meals with a high fat content disrupt the MMC with little change in gastrin levels. Also, patients with a gastrin-secreting tumour have normal MMC activity.

Thus, while gastrin may not necessarily be responsible for the initiation and maintenance of postprandial activity, together with other hormones it may in part regulate the levels of motility seen with meals of different composition.

Intestinal phase

The arrival of nutrients in the small intestine is a powerful stimulus of postprandial motor activity. Bypassing cephalic and gastric influences by introducing nutrients directly into the duodenum initiates motor patterns typical of the postprandial state. Any fluid which deviates appreciably from neutrality or osmolarity, or which contains digestion products results in the change from fasted to fed motility (see Weisbrodt, 1981).

Both local and extrinsic mechanisms are important in the intestinal phase as indicated by perfusion experiments on loops on intestine isolated from the rest of the small bowel. Perfusion of a jejunal Thiry–Vella loop with duodenal chyme collected from a donor dog initiated postprandial motor activity in both the loop and the main bowel (Figure 10.4) indicating that neural reflexes and/or hormonal mechanisms are initiated by chyme in the jejunum. Postprandial motility is similarly initiated in the Thiry–Vella loop when food is in contact with the main bowel.

CCK is one possible hormonal candidate. Like gastrin, CCK stimulates motility of a similar pattern to the postprandial pattern but again these effects are, in the main, on proximal regions with the distal small intestine being relatively 'immune' to this and other hormones.

CONCLUSION

The experiments described above would indicate that the change from

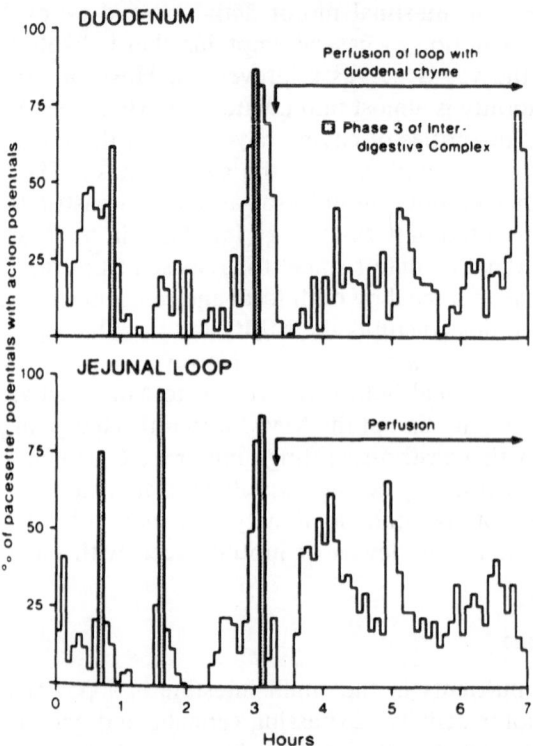

GASTROINTESTINAL MOTILITY

Figure 10.4 The effect of perfusion of a jejunal Thiry–Vella loop with duodenal chyme (collected from a donor dog) on myoelectrical activity in the duodenum and in the loop itself (From Heppell *et al.*, 1983, with kind permission of the authors and the editor of Am. J. Physiol.)

fasted to fed motor patterns is brought about by a variety of interacting factors. Extrinsic nerves are important for the immediate response to eating seen throughout the stomach and intestine and for mediating changes in motility at loci distant from the site of stimulation. Local mechanisms bring about the maintained phase of increased motor activity, and these together with a combination of hormones and extrinsic reflexes set the level of motility appropriate to the needs of digestion. Since all these processes are regulated by the volume of chyme and its composition, the reduction in these as digestion proceeds allows the restraint on the MMC to be lifted and the interdigestive pattern to resume.

References

(1) Abe, Y. and Tomita, T. (1968). Cable properties of smooth muscle. *J. Physiol. (London)*, **214**, 87–100

(2) Abrahamsson, H. (1974). Reflex adrenergic inhibition of gastric motility elicited from the gastric antrum. *Acta Physiol. Scand.*, **90**, 14–24

(3) Abrahammson, H., Glise, H. and Glise, K. (1979). Reflex suppression of gastric motility during laparotomy and gastroduodenal nociceptive stimulation. *Scand. J. Gastroenterol.*, **14**, 101–6

(4) Abrahamsson, H. and Jansson, G. (1973). Vago-vagal gastro-gastric relaxation in the cat. *Acta Physiol. Scand.*, **88**, 289–95

(5) Abrahamsson, H., Jansson, G. and Martinson, J. (1973). Vagal relaxations of the stomach induced by apomorphine in the cat. *Acta Physiol. Scand.*, **88**, 296–302

(6) Agostoni, E., Chinnock, J.E., de Burgh Daly, M. and Murray, J.G. (1957). Functional and histological studies of the vagus nerve and its branches to the heart, lungs and abdominal viscera in the cat. *J. Physiol. (London)*, **135**, 182–206

(7) Aidley, D.J. (1978). *Physiology of Excitable Cells.* 2nd Edn. (Cambridge: Cambridge University Press)

(8) Alvarez, W.C. (1939). *An Introduction to Gastroenterology.* 3rd. Edn. (London: Heinemann)

(9) Alvarez, W.C. and Mahoney, L.J. (1922). Action currents in stomach and intestine. *Am. J. Physiol.*, **58**, 476–93

(10) Andrew, B.L. (1956). The nervous control of cervical oesophagus of the rat. *J. Physiol. (London)*, **134**, 729–40

(11) Andrews, P.L.R. and Grundy, D. (1981). The effect of stimulus characteristics on the rebound contraction in the gastric corpus. *J. Physiol. (London)*, **313**, 24–25P

(12) Andrews, P.L.R., Grundy, D. and Lawes, I.N.C. (1980). The role of the vagus and splanchnic nerves in the regulation of intragastric pressure in the ferret. *J. Physiol. (London)*, **307**, 401–11

(13) Andrews, P.L.R., Grundy, D. and Scratcherd, T. (1980a). Reflex excitation of antral motility induced by gastric distension in the ferret. *J. Physiol. (London)*, **298**, 79–84

(14) Andrews, P.L.R., Grundy, D. and Scratcherd, T. (1980b). Vagal afferent discharge from mechanoreceptors in different regions of the ferret stomach. *J. Physiol. (London)*, **298**, 513–24

(15) Andrews, P.L.R. and Lawes, I.N.C. (1984). Interactions between splanchnic and vagus nerves in the control of mean intragastric pressure in the ferret. *J. Physiol. (London)*, **351**, 473–90

(16) Baumgarten, H.G. (1982). Morphological basis of gastrointestinal motility: structure and innervation of gastrointestinal tract. In Bertaccini, G. (ed.). *Mediators and Drugs in Gastrointestinal Motility I.* pp. 7–53. (Berlin: Springer–Verlag)

(17) Bayliss, W.M. and Starling, E.H. (1899). The movements and innervation of the small intestine. *J. Physiol. (London)*, **24**, 99–143

(18) Bennet, M.R., Burnstock, G. and Holman, M.E. (1966a). Transmission from perivascular inhibitory nerves to the smooth muscle of the guinea-pig taenia coli. *J. Physiol. (London)*, **182**, 527–40

(19) Bennet, M.R., Burnstock, G. and Holman, M.E. (1966b). Transmission from intramural inhibitory nerves to the smooth muscle of the guinea-pig taenia coli. *J. Physiol. (London),* **182**, 541–58

(20) Bertaccini, G. (1982). Endogenous substances which can affect gastrointestinal motility. In Bertaccini, G. (ed.). *Mediators and Drugs in Gastrointestinal Motility II.* pp. 1–10. (Berlin: Springer–Verlag)

(21) Bolton, T.B. (1979). Cholinergic mechanisms in smooth muscle. *Br. Med. Bull.,* **35**, 275–83

(22) Boldyreff, W.N. (1905). Le travail periodique de l'appareil digestif en dehors de la digestion. *Arch. Des. Sci. Biol.,* **11**, 1–157

(23) Bornstein, J.C., Costa, M., Furness, J.B. and Lees, G.M. (1984). Electrophysiology and enkephalin immunoreactivity of identified myenteric plexus neurones of guinea-pig small intestine. *J. Physiol. (London),* **351**, 313–26

(24) Bortoff, A. (1983). Smooth muscle of the gastrointestinal tract. In Christensen, J. and Wingate, D.L. (eds.). *A Guide to Gastrointestinal Motility.* pp. 48–74. (Bristol: John Wright and Sons Ltd.)

(25) Bozler, E. (1939). Electrophysiological studies on the motility of the gastrointestinal tract. *Am. J. Physiol.,* **127**, 301–7

(26) Brown, J.C., Cook, M.A. and Dryburgh, J.R. (1973). Motilin, a gastric motor activity stimulating polypeptide: the complete amino acid sequence. *Can. J. Biochem.,* **51**, 533–7

(27) Brink, B.M., Schlegal J.F. and Code, C.F. (1965). The pressure profile of the gastroduodenal junctional zone in dogs. *Gut,* **6**, 163–71

(28) Bueno, L. and Fioramonti, J. (1981). Patterns of colonic motility. In Read, N.W. (ed.). *Diarrhoea: New Insights. Clin. Res. Rev.,* **1** (Suppl. 1), 91–100

(29) Bueno, L., Fioramonti, J., Ruckebusch, Y. (1975). Rate of flow of digesta and electrical activity of the small intestine in dogs and sheep. *J. Physiol. (London),* **249**, 69–85

(30) Bueno, L., Fioramonti, J., Ruckebusch, Y., Frexinos, J. and Coulom, P. (1980). Evaluation of colonic myoelectrical acivity in health and functional disorders. *Gut,* **21**, 480–5

(31) Bueno, L., Praddaude, F. and Ruckebusch, Y. (1979). Propogation of electrical spiking activity along the small intestine: intrinsic versus extrinsic neural influences. *J. Physiol. (London),* **292**, 15–26

(32) Burnstock, G. (1975). Ultrastructure of autonomic nerves and neuroeffector junctions: analysis of drug action. In Daniel, E.E. and Paton, D.M. (eds.). *Methods in Pharmacology, Vol.III. Smooth Muscle.* pp. 113–37. (New York and London: Plenum)

(33) Burnstock, G. (1979). Autonomic innervation and transmission. *Br. Med. Bull.,* **35**, 255–62

(34) Burnstock, G. (1981). Neurotransmitters and trophic factors in the autonomic nervous system. *J. Physiol. (London),* **313**, 1–35

(35) Cambell, G.R., Uehara, Y., Monk, G. and Burnstock, G. (1971). Fine structure of smooth muscle cells grown in tissue culture. *J. Cell Biol.,* **49**, 21–34

(36) Cann, P.A. and Read, N.W. (1981). Intestinal transit and bowel disturbance. In Read, N.W. (ed.). *Diarrhoea: New Insights. Clin. Res. Rev.,* **1** (Suppl. 1), 101–5

(37) Cannon, W.B. (1902). The movements of the intestines studied by means of the Rontgen rays. *Am. J. Physiol.,* **6**, 251–77

(38) Cannon, W.B. and Lieb, C.M. (1911). The receptive relaxation of the stomach. *Am. J. Physiol.,* **29**, 270–3

(39) Caprilli, R., Frieri, G. and Vernia, P. (1982). Electrophysiology of intestinal smooth muscle. In Bertaccini, G. (ed.). *Mediators and Drugs in Gastrointestinal Motility I.* pp. 117–43. (Berlin: Springer–Verlag)

(40) Carlson, A.J. (1916). *The Control of Hunger in Health and Disease.* (Chicago: The University of Chicago Press)

(41) Carlson, G.M., Bedi, B.S. and Code, C.F. (1972). Mechanism of propagation of intestinal interdigestive myoelectric complex. *Am. J. Physiol.,* **222**, 1027–30

(42) Casteels, R. (1969). Calculation of the membrane potential in smooth muscle cells of the guinea-pig's taenia coli by the Goldman equation. *J. Physiol. (London),* **271**, 41–61

(43) Cervero, F. (1983). Somatic and visceral inputs to the thoracic spinal cord of the cat: effects of noxious stimulation of the biliary system. *J. Physiol. (London),* **337**, 51–67

REFERENCES

(44) Christensen, J. (1981). Motility of the colon. In Johnson, L.R. (ed.). *Physiology of the Gastrointestinal Tract.* pp. 445–71. (New York: Raven Press)

(45) Christensen, J. (1983). The oesophagus. In Christensen, J. and Wingate, D.L. (eds.). *A Guide to Gastrointestinal Motility.* pp. 75–100. (Bristol: John Wright and Sons Ltd.)

(46) Christensen, J., Anuras, S. and Hauser, R. L. (1974). Migrating spike bursts and electrical slow waves in the cat colon: effect of sectioning. *Gastroenterology, 66,* 240–7

(47) Clarke, G.D. and Davison, J.S. (1976). Response of distension sensitive vagal afferent nerve endings to controlled inflation of the rat stomach. *J. Physiol. (London), 256,* 122–3P

(48) Cocks, T. and Burnstock, G. (1979). Effects of neuronal polypeptides on intestinal smooth muscle: a comparison with non-adrenergic, non-cholinergic nerve stimulation and ATP. *Eur. J. Pharmacol., 54,* 251–9

(49) Code, C.F. and Marlett, J. A. (1975). The interdigestive myoelectric complex of the stomach and small bowel of dogs. *J. Physiol. (London), 246,* 289–309

(50) Code, C.F. and Schlegel, J.F. (1974). The gastrointestinal interdigestive housekeeper: Motor correlates of the interdigestive myoelectric complex of the dog. In *Proceeding of the IVth International Symposium on Gastrointestinal Motility.* Daniel, E. E. (ed.). pp. 631–3. (Vancouver: Mitchell Press)

(51) Collman, P.I., Grundy, D. and Scratcherd, T. (1983). Vagal influences on the jejunal minute rhythm in the anaesthetized ferret. *J. Physiol. (London), 345,* 65–74

(52) Collman, P.I., Grundy, D. and Scratcherd, T. (1984a). Vagal control of colonic motility in the anaesthetized ferret: evidence for a non-cholinergic excitatory innervation. *J. Physiol. (London), 348,* 35–42

(53) Collman, P.I., Grundy, D. and Scratcherd, T. (1984b). Vagal and splanchnic influences on small intestinal motility in the anaesthetized ferret. In Roman, C. (ed.). *Gastrointestinal Motility: Proceedings of the 9th International Symposium on Gastrointestinal Motility.* pp. 373–80. (Lancaster: MTP Press)

(54) Collman, P.I., Grundy, D., Scratcherd, T. and Wach, R.A. (1984c). Vago-vagal reflexes to the colon of the anaesthetized ferret. *J. Physiol. (London), 352,* 395–402

(55) Cohen, S. and Harris, L.D. (1976). Anatomy and normal functional physiology of the esophagus and pharynx. In Dietschy, J.M. (ed.). *Disorders of the Gastrointestinal Tract: Disorders of the Liver and Nutritional Disorders.* pp. 1–3. (New York, Grune and Stratton)

(56) Cooke, A.R. (1975). Control of gastric emptying and motility. *Gastroenterology, 68,* 804–16

(57) Costa, M. and Furness, J.B. (1976). The peristaltic reflex: An analysis of the nerve pathways and their pharmacology. *Naunyn-Schmiedberg's. Arch. Pharmacol., 294,* 47–60

(58) Costa, M. and Furness, J.B. (1982). Nervous control of intestinal motility. In Bertaccini, G. (ed.). *Mediators and Drugs in Gastrointestinal Motility I.* pp. 279–382. (Berlin: Springer–Verlag)

(59) Daniel, E.E. (1982). Pharmacology of adrenergic, cholinergic, and drugs acting on other receptors in gastrointestinal muscle. In Bertaccini, G. (ed.). *Mediators and Drugs in Gastrointestinal Motility II.* pp. 248–322. (Berlin: Springer–Verlag)

(60) Davison, J.S. (1972). Response of single vagal afferent fibres to mechanical and chemical stimulation of the gastric and duodenal mucosa in cats. *Q. J. Exp. Physiol., 57,* 405–16

(61) Davison, J.S. (1983). Innervation of the gastrointestinal tract. In Christensen, J. and Wingate, D.L. (eds.). *A Guide to Gastrointestinal Motility.* pp. 1–47. (Bristol: John Wright and Sons Ltd.)

(62) Davison, J.S., Gradwell, D.P. and Hersteinsson, P. (1977). Synapsing pathways through the guinea-pig inferior mesenteric ganglia. *Experientia, 33,* 610–1

(63) Davison, J. and Grundy, D. (1978). Modulation of single vagal efferent fibre discharge by gastrointestinal afferents in the rat. *J. Physiol. (London), 284,* 69–82

(64) Defilippi, C. and Valenzuela, J.E. (1981). Sham feeding disrupts the interdigestive motility complex in man. *Scand. J. Gastroenterol., 16,* 977–80

(65) De Groat, W.C. and Krier, J. (1978). The sacral reflex pathway regulating colonic motility and defecation in the cat. *J. Physiol. (London), 276,* 481–500

171

(66) Diamant, N.E. and Bortoff, A. (1969a). Nature of the intestinal slow-wave frequency gradient. *Am. J. Physiol.*, **216**, 301–7
(67) Diamant, N.E. and Bortoff, A. (1969b). Effects of transection on the intestinal slow-wave frequency gradient. *Am. J. Physiol.*, **216**, 734–43
(68) Diamant, N.E., Hall, K., Mui, H. and El-Sharkawy, T.Y. (1980). Vagal control of the feeding motor pattern in the lower esophageal sphincter, stomach, and small intestine of dog. In Christensen, J. (ed.). *Gastrointestinal Motility*. pp. 365–70. (New York: Raven Press)
(69) Diamant, N.E. and El-Sharkawy, T.Y. (1977). Neural control of esophageal peristalsis: a conceptual analysis. *Gastroenterology*, **72**, 546–56
(70) Dockray, G.J and Gregory, R.A. (1980). Relations between neuropeptides and gut hormones. *Proc. R. Soc. London (B)*, **210** (No. 1178), 151–64
(71) Dodds, W.J., Christensen, J., Dent, J., Wood, J.D and Arndorfer, R.C. (1978). Esophagus contractions induced by vagal stimulation in the opossum. *Am. J. Physiol.*, **235**, E392–401
(72) Edin, R. (1980). The vagal control of the pyloric motor function: a physiological and immunohistochemical study in cat and man. *Acta Physiol. Scand.* (Suppl), **485**, 1–30
(73) Ehrlein, H.J. and Akkermans, L.M.A. (1984). Gastric emptying. In Akkermans, L.M.A, Johnson, A.G.and Read, N.W. (eds.). *Gastric and Gastroduodenal Motility*. pp. 74–86. (Eastbourne: Praeger)
(74) Ehrlein, H.J., Keinke, 0. and Schemann, M. (1984). Studies on the process of gastric emptying. In Roman, C. (ed.). *Gastrointestinal Motility: Proceedings of the 9th International Symposium on Gastrointestinal Motility*. pp. 111–8. (Lancaster: MTP Press)
(75) Ehrlein, H.-J., Reich, H. and Schwinger, M. (1982). Physiological significance of the contractions the rabbit proximal colon. *Q. J. Exp. Physiol.*, **67**, 407–17
(76) Eklund, S., Jodel, M., Lundgren, O. and Sjoqvist, A. (1979). Effects of vasoactive intestinal polypeptide on blood flow, motility, and fluid transport in the gastrointestinal tract of the cat. *Acta Physiol. Scand.*, **105**, 461–8
(77) Eliasson, S. (1960). Central control of digestive function. In Field, J. (ed.-in-chief). *Handbook of Physiology, Sect.1, Vol. II*. pp. 1163–72. (Washington, D.C.: American Physiological Society)
(78) Fahrenkrug, J., Haglund, U., Jodal, M., Lundgren, O., Olbe, L. and Schaffalitzky-De-Muckadell, O.B. (1978). Nervous release of vasoactive intestinal polypeptide in the gastrointestinal tract of cats: Possible physiological implications. *J. Physiol. (London)*, **284**, 291–305
(79) Falempin, M. and Rousseau, J.P. (1984). Effects of the vagal deafferentation on oesophageal motility in the conscious sheep. In Roman, C. (ed.). Gastrointestinal Motility: Proceedings of the 9th International Symposium on Gastrointestinal Motility. pp. 3–8. (Lancaster: MTP Press)
(80) Fasth, S., Hulten, L. and Nordgren, S. (1980). Evidence for a dual pelvic nerve influence on large bowel motility in the cat. *J. Physiol. (London)*, **298**, 159–69
(81) Fleckenstein, P., Bueno, L., Fioramonti, J. and Ruckebusch, Y. (1982). Minute rhythm of electrical spike bursts of the small intestine in different species. *Am. J. Physiol.*, **242**, G654–9
(82) Fleckenstein, P., Oigaard, A. (1978). Electrical spike activity in the human small intestine. A multiple electrode study of fasting diurnal variations. *Dig. Dis. Sci.*, **23**, 776–80
(83) Furness, J.B., Cambell, G.R., Gillard, S.M., Malmfors, T., Cobb, J.L.S. and Burnstock, G. (1970). Cellular studies of sympathetic denervation produced by 6-hydroxydopamine in the vas deferens. *J. Pharm. Exp. Ther.*, **174**, 111–22
(84) Gabella, G. (1976). *Structure of the Autonomic Nervous System*. (London: Chapman and Hall)
(85) Gabella, G. (1979a). Smooth muscle cell junctions and structural aspects of contraction. *Br Med. Bull.*, **35**, 213–8
(86) Gabella, G. (1979b). Innervation of the gastrointestinal tract. *Int. Rev. Cytochem.*, **59**, 129–93
(87) Gabella, G. (1981). Structure of muscle and nerves in the gastrointestinal tract. In Johnson, L.R. (ed.). *Physiology of the Gastrointestinal Tract Vol 1*. pp. 197–241. (New York: Raven Press)

REFERENCES

(88) Garnier, L. and Mei, N. (1982). Do true osmoreceptors exist at intestinal level? *J. Physiol. (London)*, **327**, 97P–8P

(89) Gonella, J., Niel, J.P. and Roman, C. (1977). Vagal control of lower oesophageal sphincter motility in the cat. *J. Physiol. (London)*, **273**, 647–64

(90) Gonella, J., Niel, J.P. and Roman, C. (1979). Sympathetic control of lower oeso-phageal sphincter motility in the cat. *J. Physiol. (London)*, **287**, 177–90

(91) Gonella, J., Niel, J.P. and Roman, C. (1980). Mechanism of the noradrenergic motor control of the lower oesophageal sphincter motility in the cat. *J. Physiol. (London)*, **306**, 251–60

(92) Goyal, R.K. (1978). Neurology of the gut. In Sleisenger, M.H. and Fordtran, J.S. (eds.). *Gastrointestinal Disease. Pathophysiology, Diagnosis, Management.* pp. 156–78. (Philadelphia: W.B. Saunders Co.)

(93) Goyal, R.K. and Cobb, B.W. (1981). Motility of the pharynx, esophagus, and eso-phageal sphincters. In Johnson, L.R. (ed.). *Physiology of the Gastrointestinal Tract Vol 1*. pp. 359–91. (New York: Raven Press)

(94) Goyal, R.K., Said, S. and Rattan, S. (1979). Influence of VIP antiserum on lower esophageal sphincter relaxation: possible evidence for VIP as the inhibitory transmitter. *Gastroenterology*, **76**, 1142

(95) Gregory, R.A. (1950). Some factors influencing the passage of fluid through intestinal loops in dogs. *J. Physiol. (London)*, **111**, 119–37

(96) Grivel, M.-L. and Ruckebusch, Y. (1972). The propogation of segmental contractions along the small intestine. *J. Physiol. (London)*, **227**, 611–25

(97) Grundy, D., Salih, A.A. and Scratcherd, T. (1981). Modulation of vagal efferent discharge by mechanoreceptors in the stomach, duodenum and colon of the ferret. *J. Physiol. (London)*, **319**, 43–52

(98) Grundy, D. and Scratcherd, T. (1982). A splanchno-vagal component of the inhibition of gastric motility by distension of the intestines. In Wienbeck, M. (ed.). *Motility of the Digestive Tract.* pp. 39–43. (New York: Raven Press)

(99) Grundy, D. and Scratcherd, T. (1984). The role of the vagus and sympathetic nerves in the control of gastric motility. In Akkermans, L.M.A, Johnson, A.G.and Read, N.W. (eds.). *Gastric and Gastroduodenal Motility.* pp. 21–33. (Eastbourne: Praeger)

(100) Hall, K. E., El-Sharkawy, T. Y. and Diamant, N. E. (1982). Vagal control of migrating motor complex in the dog. *Am. J. Physiol.*, **243**, G276–84

(101) Hall, K. E., Greenberg, G. E., El-Sharkawy, T.Y. and Diamant, N. E. (1983). Vagal control of migrating motor complex-related peaks in canine plasma motilin, pancreatic polypeptide and gastrin. *Can. J. Physiol. Pharmacol.*, **61**, 1289–98

(102) Halls, J. (1965). Bowel content shift during normal defaecation. *Proc. R. Soc. Med.*, **58**, 859–60

(103) Harding, R. and Leek, B.F. (1972). The effects of peripheral and central nervous influences on gastric centre neuronal activity in sheep. *J. Physiol. (London)*, **225**, 309–38

(104) Harper, A.A., Kidd, C. and Scratcherd, T. (1959). Vago-vagal reflex effects on gastric and pancreatic secretion and gastrointestinal motility. *J. Physiol. (London)*, **148**, 417–36

(105) Hartshorne, D.J. (1981). Biochemistry of the contractile process in smooth muscle. In Johnson, L.R. (ed.). *Physiology of the Gastrointestinal Tract Vol 1*. pp. 243–67. (New York: Raven Press)

(106) Heading, R.C., Logan, R.F.A., Mcloughlin, G.P., Lidgard, G. and Forrest, J.A.H. (1977). Effect of cimetidine on gastric emptying. In Burland, W.L. and Simkins, M.A. (eds.). *Cimetidine: Proceedings of the 2nd International Symposium on Histamine H₂-Receptor Antagonists*. pp. 145–52. (Amsterdam and Oxford: Excerpta Medica)

(107) Heppell, J., Becker, J.M., Kelly, K.A. and Zinsmeister, A.R. (1983). Postprandial inhibition of canine enteric interdigestive myoelectric complex. *Am. J. Physiol.*, **244**, G160–4

(108) Heppell, J., Kelly, K.A. and Sarr, M.G. (1983). Neural control of canine small intestinal interdigestive myoelectric complexes. *Am. J. Physiol.*, **244**, G95–100

(109) Hirst, G.D.S., Holman, M.E. and McKirdy, H.C. (1975). Two descending nerve pathways activated by distension of guinea-pig small intestine. *J. Physiol. (London)*, **244**, 113–27

(110) Hirst, G.D.S, Holman, M.E. and Spence, I. (1974). Two types of neurone in the myenteric plexus of duodenum in the guinea-pig. *J. Physiol. (London)*, **236**, 303–26

(111) Hirst, G.D.S. and McKirdy, H.C. (1974). A nervous mechanism for descending inhibition in guinea-pig small intestine. *J. Physiol. (London)*, **238**, 129–43

(112) Hodgkiss, J.P. and Lees, G.M. (1980). Morphological features of guinea-pig myenteric plexus neurones. In Christensen, J. (ed.). *Gastrointestinal Motility*. pp. 111–8. (New York: Raven Press)

(113) Hokfelt, T., Johansson, O., Ljungdahl, A., Lundberg, J.M. and Schultzberg, M. (1980). Peptidergic neurones. *Nature*, **284**, 515–21

(114) Holman, M.E. and Neild, T.O. (1979). Membrane properties. *Br. Med. Bull.*, **35**, 235–41

(115) Hunt, J.N. and Knox, M.T. (1968). Regulation of gastric emptying. In Code, C.F. and Heidel, W. (eds.). *Handbook of Physiology, Section 6, Vol. 4, Alimentary Canal*. pp. 1917–35. (Washington D.C.: American Physiological Society)

(116) Hunt, J.N. and Macdonald, I. (1954). The influence of gastric volume on gastric emptying. *J. Physiol. (London)*, **126**, 459–74

(117) Hunt, J.N. and Stubbs, D.F. (1975). The volume and energy content of meals as determinants of gastric emptying. *J. Physiol. (London)*, **215**, 209–25

(118) Iggo, A. (1955). Tension receptors in the stomach and the urinary bladder. *J. Physiol. (London)*, **128**, 593–607

(119) Itoh, Z., Honda, R, Hiwatashi, K., Aizawa, I., Takayanagi, R. and Couch, E.F. (1976). Motilin-induced mechanical activity in the canine alimentary tract. *Scand. J. Gastroenterol.*, **11** (Suppl. 39), 93–110

(120) Itoh, Z. and Sekiguchi, T. (1982). Interdigestive motor activity in health and disease. *Scand. J. Gastroenterol.*, **18** (Suppl. 82), 497–521

(121) Jahnberg, T., Abrahamsson, H., Jansson, G. and Martinson, J. (1977). Gastric relaxatory response to feeding before and after vagotomy. *Scand. J. Gastroenterol.*, **12**, 225–8

(122) Jansson, G. and Martinson, J. (1966). Studies on the ganglionic site of action of the sympathetic outflow to the stomach. *Acta Physiol. Scand.*, **68**, 184–92

(123) Jeanningros, R. (1982). Vagal unitary responses to intestinal amino acid infusions in the anaesthetized cat: a putative signal for protein induced satiety. *Physiol. Behav.*, **28**, 9–21

(124) Jeanningros, R. (1984). Modulation of lateral hypothalamic single unit activity by gastric and intestinal distension. *J. Autonom. Nerv. Syst.*, **11**, 1–13

(125) Kelly, K.A. (1976). Gastric motility in health and after gastric surgery. *Viewpoints Dig. Dis.*, **8**, 1–4

(126) Kelly, K.A. (1981). Motility of the stomach and gastroduodenal junction. In Johnson, L.R. (ed.). *Physiology of the Gastrointestinal Tract Vol 1*. pp. 393–410. (New York: Raven Press)

(127) Kelly, K.A., Code, C.F. and Elveback, L.R. (1969). Patterns of canine gastric electrical activity. *Am. J. Physiol.*, **217**, 461–70

(128) King, B.F. and Szurszewski, J.H. (1984). Intracellular recordings from vagally innervated intramural neurones in opossum stomach. *Am. J. Physiol.*, **246**, G209–12

(129) King, B.F. and Szurszewski, J.H. (1984). Mechanoreceptor pathways from the distal colon to the autonomic nervous system in the guinea-pig. *J. Physiol. (London)*, **350**, 93–108

(130) Konturek, S.J. (1984). Gastrointestinal hormones and intestinal motility. In Roman, C. (ed.). *Gastrointestinal Motility: Proceedings of the 9th International Symposium on Gastrointestinal Motility*. pp. 593–612. (Lancaster: MTP Press)

(131) Kreulen, D. L. and Szurszewski, J. H. (1979). Reflex pathways in the abdominal prevertebral ganglia: evidence for a colo-colonic inhibitory reflex. *J. Physiol. (London)*, **295**, 21–32

(132) Langley, J.N. (1921). *The Autonomic Nervous System. Part 1*. (Cambridge: W. Heffer and Sons)

(133) Leek, B.F. (1977). Abdominal and pelvic visceral receptors. *Br. Med. Bull.*, **33**, 163–8

(134) Malmud, L.S., Fisher, R.S., Knight, L.C. and Rock, E. (1982). Scintigraphic evaluation of gastric emptying. *Seminars in Nuclear Medicine*, **XII** (no. 2), 116–25

(135) Mamber, L. and Gershon, M.D. (1979). A reciprocal adrenergic–cholinergic axoaxonic synapse in the mammalian gut. *Am. J. Physiol.*, **236**, E738–45

REFERENCES

(136) Mei, N. (1978). Vagal glucoreceptors in the small intestine of the cat. *J. Physiol. (London)*, **282**, 485–506

(137) Mei, N. (1983). Recent studies on intestinal vagal afferent innervation. Functional implications. *J. Autonom. Nerv. Syst.*, **9**, 199–206

(138) Miolan J.P. and Roman, C. (1974). Decharge unitaire des fibres vagales efferentes lors de la relaxation receptive de l'estomac du chien. *J. Physiol. (Paris)*, **68**, 693–704

(139) Miolan J.P. and Roman, C. (1978a). Activite des fibres vagales efferentes destinees a la musculature lisse du cardia du chien. *J. Physiol. (Paris)*, **74**, 709–23

(140) Miolan, J. P. and Roman, C. (1978b). Discharge of efferent vagal fibers supplying gastric antrum: indirect study by nerve suture technique. *Am. J. Physiol.*, **235**, E366–73

(141) Morita, K., Katayama, Y. and North, R.A. (1980). Chymotrypsin attenuates synaptic potentials: evidence that substance P is a neurotransmitter within the myenteric plexus. *Nature*, **287**, 151–2

(142) Morrison, J.F.B. (1977). The afferent innervation of the gastrointestinal tract. In Brooks, F.B. and Evers, P.W. (eds.). *Nerves and the Gut.* pp. 297–326. (New Jersey: C.B.S.)

(143) Nishi, S. and North, R.A. (1973). Intracellular recordings from the myenteric plexus of the guinea-pig ileum. *J. Physiol. (London)*, **231**, 471–91

(144) Norberg, K.A. (1964). Adrenergic innervation of the intestinal wall studied by fluorescence microscopy. *Int. J. Neuropharmacol.*, **3**, 379–82

(145) North, R.A. (1982). Electrophysiology of the enteric neurons In Bertaccini, G. (ed.). *Mediators and Drugs in Gastrointestinal Motility I.* pp. 145–79. (Berlin: Springer–Verlag)

(146) Pahlin, P.-E. and Kewenter, J. (1975). Reflexogenic contractions of the ileocecal sphincter in the cat following small or large intestinal distension. *Acta Physiol. Scand.*, **95**, 126–32

(147) Pahlin, P.-E. and Kewenter, J. (1976a). Sympathetic nervous control of the cat ileocecal sphincter. *Am. J. Physiol.*, **231**, 296–305

(148) Pahlin, P.-E. and Kewenter, J. (1976b). The vagal control of the ileocecal sphincter in the cat. *Acta Physiol. Scand.*, **96**, 433–42

(149) Peeters, T.L., Janssens, J. and Vantrappen, G.R. (1983). Somatostatin and the interdigestive migrating motor complex in man. *Regul. Peptides*, **5**, 209–17

(150) Peeters, T.L., Vantrappen, G.R. and Janssens, J. (1982). Control of gut motility. In Bloom, S.R., Polak, J.M. and Lindenlaub, E. (eds.). *Systemic Role of Regulatory Peptides.* pp. 194–208. (Stuttgart–New York: F.K. Schattauer Verlag)

(151) Prove, J. and Ehrlein, H.J. (1982). Motor function of gastric antrum and pylorus for evacuation of low and high viscosity meals in dogs. *Gut*, **23**, 150–6

(152) Read, N.W., McFarlane, A., Kinsman, R.I. and Bloom, S.R. (1984). The ileal brake: a potent mechanism for feedback control of gastric emptying and small bowel transit. In Roman, C. (ed.). *Gastrointestinal Motility: Proceedings of the 9th International Symposium on Gastrointestinal Motility.* pp. 335–42. (Lancaster: MTP Press)

(153) Renny, A., Snape, W.J., Sun, E.A., London, R. and Cohen, S. (1983). Role of cholecystokinin in the gastro-colonic response to a fat meal. *Gastroenterology*, **85**, 17–21

(154) Roman, C. and Gonella, J. (1981). Extrinsic control of digestive tract motility. In Johnson, L.R. (ed.). *Physiology of the Gastrointestinal Tract Vol 1.* pp. 289–333. (New York: Raven Press)

(155) Roman, C. and Tieffenbach, L. (1972). Enregistrement de l'activite unitaire des fibres motrices vagales destinees a l'oesophage du babouin. *J. Physiol. (Paris)*, **64**, 479–506

(156) Ruckebusch, Y. and Bueno, L. (1976). The effect of feeding on the motility of the stomach and small intestine in the pig. *Br. J. Nutr.*, **35**, 397–405

(157) Ruckebusch, Y. and Bueno, L. (1977). Migrating myoelectrical complex of the small intestine. An intrinsic activity mediated by the vagus. *Gastroenterology*, **73**, 1309–14

(158) Ruckebusch, Y. and Fioramonti, J. (1980). Colonic myoelectric spiking activity: major patterns and significance in six different species. *Zentralblatt fur Veterinarmedizin A*, **27**, 1–8

(159) Ruckebusch, Y., Grivel, M.-L. and Fargeas, M.-J. (1971). Activite electrique de l'intestin et prise de nourriture conditionelle chez le lapin. *Physiol. Behav.*, **6**, 359–65

175

(160) Sarna, S.K., Chey, W., Condon, R., Dodds, W., Myers, T. and Chang, T. (1984). Motilin release and the migrating myoelectric complexes. In Roman, C. (ed.). *Gastrointestinal Motility: Proceedings of the 9th International Symposium on Gastrointestinal Motility.* pp. 223–30. (Lancaster: MTP Press)

(161) Sarna, S., Condon, R.E. and Cowles, V. (1983). Enteric mechanisms of initiation of migrating myoelectric complexes in dogs. *Gastroenterology,* **84**, 814–22

(162) Sarna, S., Northcott, P. and Belbeck, L. (1982). Mechanisms of cycling of migrating myoelectric complexes: effect of morphine. *Am. J. Physiol.,* **242**, G588–95

(163) Sarna, S., Stoddard, C., Belbeck, L. and Mcwade, D. (1981a). Intrinsic nervous control of migrating myoelectric complex. *Am. J. Physiol.,* **241**, G16–23

(164) Sarna, S.K., Waterfall, W.E., Bardakjian, B.L. and Lind, J.F. (1981b). Types of human colonic electrical activities recorded postoperatively. *Gastroenterology,* **81**, 61–70

(165) Sauer, M.E. and Rumble, C.T. (1946). The number of nerve cells in the myenteric and submucous plexus of the small intestine of the cat. *Anat. Rec.,* **96**, 373–81

(166) Schulze-Delrieu, K., Wright, B., Lu, C. and Shirazi, S.S. (1984). Effects of nervous stimulation on pyloric resistance and configuration. In Roman, C. (ed.). *Gastrointestinal Motility: Proceedings of the 9th International Symposium on Gastrointestinal Motility.* pp. 121–8. (Lancaster: MTP Press)

(167) Schuster, M.H., Hookman, P., Hendrix, T.R. and Mendeloff, A.I. (1965). Simultaneous manometric recording of internal and external anal sphincteric reflexes. *Bull. Johns Hopkins Hosp.,* **116**, 79–88

(168) Scratcherd, T. and Grundy, D. (1982). Nervous afferents from the upper gastrointestinal tract which influence gastrointestinal motility. In Wienbeck, M. (ed.). *Motility of the Digestive Tract.* pp. 7–16. (New York: Raven Press)

(169) Sleisenger, M.H. and Silverberg, M. (1978). The colon: anatomy and developmental anomalies. In Sleisenger, M.H. and Fordtran, J.S. (eds.). *Gastrointestinal Disease: Physiology, Diagnosis, Management.* pp. 1505–23. (Philadelphia, London, Toronto: W.B. Saunders Co

(170) Small, J.V. and Squire, J.M. (1972). Structural basis of contraction in vertebrate smooth muscle. *J. Mol. Biol.,* **67**, 117–49

(171) Snape, W.J., Wright, S.H., Battle, W.M. and Cohen, S. (1979). The gastrocolic reflex: evidence for a neural mechanism. *Gastroenterology,* **77**, 1235–40

(172) Solcia, E., Capella, C., Buffa, R., Usellini, L., Fiocca, R. and Sessa, F. (1981). Endocrine cells of the digestive system. In Johnson, L.R. (ed.). *Physiology of the Gastrointestinal Tract Vol 1.* pp. 39–58. (New York: Raven Press)

(173) Summers, R.W. and Dusdieker, N.S. (1980). Computer-generated display of longitudinal spike burst spread in the small intestine. In Christensen, J. (ed.). *Gastrointestinal Motility.* pp. 339–44. (New York: Raven Press)

(174) Summers, R.W, Kent, T.H. and Osborne, J.W. (1970). Effects of drugs, ileal obstruction, and irradiation on rat gastrointestinal propulsion. *Gastroenterology,* **59**, 731–9

(175) Szurszewski, J.H. (1969). A migrating electric complex of the canine small intestine. *Am. J. Physiol.,* **217**, 1757–63

(176) Szurszewski, J.H. (1977a). Towards a new view of prevertebral ganglion. In Brooks, F.B. and Evers, P.W. (eds.). *Nerves and the Gut.* pp. 244–60. (New Jersey: C.B.S.)

(177) Szurszewski, J.H. (1977b). Modulation of smooth muscle by nervous activity: a review and a hypothesis. *Fed. Proc.,* **36**, 2456–61

(178) Szurszewski, J.H. (1981a). Electrophysiological basis for gastrointestinal motility. In Johnson, L.R. (ed.). *Physiology of the Gastrointestinal Tract Vol 2.* pp. 1435–66. (New York: Raven Press)

(179) Szurszewski, J.H. (1981b). Physiology of mammalian prevertebral ganglia. *Annu. Rev. Physiol.,* **43**, 53–68

(180) Templeton, R.D. and Lawson, H. (1931). Studies in the motor activity of the large intestine 1. Normal motility in the dog, recorded by the tandem balloon method. *Am. J. Physiol.,* **96**, 667–76

(181) Thomas, P.A. and Kelly, K.A. (1979). Hormonal control of interdigestive motor cycles of canine proximal stomach. *Am. J. Physiol.,* **237**, E192–7

(182) Vantrappen, G., Janssens, J., Hellemans, J. and Ghoos, Y. (1977). The interdigestive

REFERENCES

motor complex of normal subjects and patients with bacterial overgrowth of the small intestine. *J. Clin. Invest.*, **59**, 1158–66

(183) Walsh, J.H. (1981). Gastrointestinal hormones and peptides. In Johnson, L.R. (ed.). *Physiology of the Gastrointestinal Tract Vol 1*. pp. 59–144. (New York: Raven Press)

(184) Weisbrodt, N.W. (1981). Motility of the small intestine. In Johnson, L.R. (ed.). *Physiology of the Gastrointestinal Tract Vol 1*. pp. 411–43. (New York: Raven Press)

(185) Weisbrodt, N.W. and Christensen, J. (1972). Gradient of contraction in the opossum esophagus. *Gastroenterology*, **62**, 1159–66

(186) Weisbrodt, N.W., Copeland, E.M., Thor, P.I. and Dudrick, S.R. (1976). The myoelectric activity of the small intestine of the dog during total parenteral nutrition. *Proc. Soc. Biol. Med.*, **153**, 121–4

(187) Wilkie, D.R. (1976). *Muscle*. 2nd Edn. (London: Edward Arnold Ltd.)

(188) Wingate, D.L. (1981). Backwards and forwards with the migrating complex. *Am. J. Dig. Dis. Sci.*, **26**, 641–66

(189) Wingate, D.L. (1983). The small intestine. In Christensen, J. and Wingate, D.L. (eds.). *A guide to Gastrointestinal Motility*. pp. 128–56. (Bristol: John Wright and Sons Ltd.)

(190) Wood, J.D. (1972). Excitation of intestinal muscle by atropine, tetrodotoxin and xylocaine. *Am. J. Physiol.*, **222**, 118–25

(191) Wood, J.D. (1975). Neurophysiology of Auerbach's plexus and control of intestinal motility. *Physiol. Rev.*, **55**, 307–24

(192) Wood, J.D. (1981). Physiology of the enteric nervous system. In Johnson, L.R. (ed.). *Physiology of the Gastrointestinal Tract Vol 1*. pp. 1–37. (New York: Raven Press)

(193) Wood, J.D. and Mayer, C.J. (1978). Electrical activity of myenteric neurones: comparison of results obtained with intracellular and extracellular methods of recording. In Duthie, H. (ed.). *Gastrointestinal Motility in Health and Disease*. pp. 311–20. (Lancaster: MTP Press)

(194) Yokoyama, S. (1971). Evoked potentials of the Auerbach's plexus in the rabbit small intestine. *Proc. Int. Union Physiol. Sci.*, **IX**, 613

Further reading

(1) Akkermans, L.M.A., Johnson, A.G. and Read, N.W. (eds.) (1984). *Gastric and Gastroduodenal Motility*. (Eastbourne, New York: Praeger)
(2) Bertaccini, G. (ed.) (1982). *Mediators and Drugs in Gastrointestinal Motility, Vols 1 and 2*. (Berlin, Heidelberg, New York: Springer–Verlag)
(3) Bulbring, E. and Bolton, T.B. (eds.) (1979). *Smooth Muscle. Br. Med. Bull.* **35**(3)
(4) Christensen, J and Wingate, D.L. (eds.) (1983). *A Guide to Gastrointestinal Motility*. (Bristol: John Wright and Sons Ltd.)
(5) Gabella, G. (1976). *Structure of the Autonomic Nervous System*. (London: Chapman and Hall)
(6) Huddart, H. and Hunt, S. (1975). *Visceral Muscle: Its Structure and Function*. (Glasgow, London: Blackie)
(7) Johnson, L.R. (ed.) (1981). *Physiology of the Gastrointestinal Tract, Vols 1 and 2*. (New York: Raven Press)
(8) Sleisenger, M.H. and Fordtran, J.S. (eds.) (1983). *Gastrointestinal Disease: Pathophysiology, Diagnosis, Management*. 3rd Edn. (Philadelphia, London, Toronto: W.B. Saunders Co.)

Index